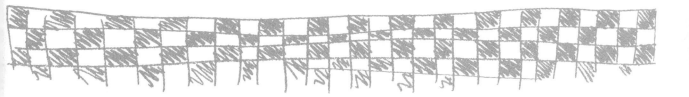

The
Arthritis Cure
Cookbook

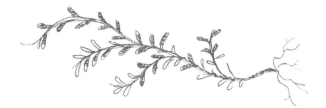

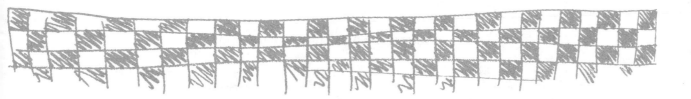

The Arthritis Cure Cookbook

By Brenda Adderly, M.H.A.
and
Lissa De Angelis, M.S., C.C.P.

LifeLine
Press

Washington, DC

Library of Congress Cataloging-in-Publication Data

Adderly, Brenda.
    The arthritis cure cookbook / by Brenda Adderly and Lissa De Angelis.
         p.   cm.
    Includes index.
    ISBN 0–89526–375–0
    1. Osteoarthritis—Diet therapy—Recipes.   I. De Angelis, Lissa.
    II. Title.
    RC931.067A33   1998
    616.7'2230654—dc21   98–4516
                                        CIP

Published in the United States by
LifeLine Press
An Eagle Publishing Company
One Massachusetts Avenue, NW
Washington, DC 20001

Distributed to the trade by
National Book Network
4720-A Boston Way
Lanham, MD 20706

Printed on acid-free paper.
Manufactured in the United States of America

Design and illustrations by Marja Walker

10 9 8 7 6 5 4 3 2 1

Books are available in quantity for promotional or premium use. Write to Director of Special Sales, LifeLine Press, One Massachusetts Avenue, NW, Washington, DC 20001, for information on discounts and terms or call (202) 216-0600.

Table of Contents

Acknowledgements

I would like to thank Howard Cohl, Mari Florence and Jeffry Still for your important contributions in making this the definitive cookbook for arthritis sufferers. Your efforts will greatly enhance the lives of millions.

—Brenda Adderly

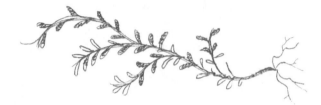

My first expression of gratitude goes to my parents, Adolph and Dorothy De Angelis, who have always encouraged and supported me. Also thank you to: my husband Cosmo Guarriello, my champion who brings all of my dreams into reality, lives life as a possibility, and shares the adventure; Helene, Bob, Joshua and Kimberly Nahm—blood for my blood for your unconditional love; my daughters Dawn, Lisa, and Jennifer, and my father-in-law, Victor, who have brought much joy and happiness to my life; my best friend Linda Dix and her husband Bruce Seiden whose compassion, friendship, and coaching go beyond all bounds; my dear friends Chris and Mark Seasly, Marie Mattie, Joan and Bob Axelrod, and Ann Nolan who authentically share life with me; Molly Siple—thanks for lighting the way to writing books, and for the many levels of work we do together; and Howard Cohl and Jeffry Still who worked with me to bring this vision to light. My heart sends all of you much appreciation for your support, encouragement, and unending belief in me.

—Lissa De Angelis

Authors' Note

Our primary goal in writing this book is to help you better understand how taking control of your nutritional needs can be a powerful tool in affecting your health. A secondary goal is to encourage you to increase the communication between yourself and your health care provider. In this context, you may choose to share this book with him or her and work together to help you achieve better health.

While this book is based on the latest scientific and dietary information about osteoarthritis, no treatment program, including drugs, nutritional supplementation, or lifestyle changes, is effective for everyone—despite promising statistics. Nothing in the content of this book is intended to suggest that the use of these dietary suggestions will fully eradicate or reverse osteoarthritis. Some people may not obtain the desired results, despite their treatment or lifestyle changes.

So, whether you have osteoarthritis or another health problem, please consult with your physician before beginning any dietary program. Because each person's biochemistry is different, the choices you make about your health should be made and applied only after consulting with your physician or other qualified health professionals. If you are taking medications, you and your physician may want to monitor your progress on this program to see if your condition improves. But please do not make any changes to your medications without first consulting your doctor. Despite your best intentions, it can be very dangerous to suddenly stop taking certain drugs.

For more information and updates on *The Arthritis Cure* and other promising health care breakthroughs, visit the author's website at www.BrendaAdderly.com.

Introducing the Arthritis Cure Diet

For the millions of Americans suffering from osteoarthritis, the solutions and suggestions provided in *The Arthritis Cure* were a welcome event. A painful and frequently debilitating disease, many American physicians previously considered osteoarthritis an inevitable byproduct of aging—incurable and treatable only with harsh drugs.

Today we know that the symptoms of arthritis can be greatly alleviated or even reversed by two commonly used natural substances: glucosamine and chondroitin sulfates. While this information has been widely understood in many other countries around the globe, its implementation in the United States had been slow to take root, until the overwhelming success of *The Arthritis Cure* brought this information into the layperson's household.

The facts about this treatment are amazing. First, and most importantly, the "cure" can be found, without a prescription, in most health food stores in America. Second, because both these compounds are made up of substances our bodies already use, there are no known side effects. This is particularly noteworthy because the other treatments for osteoarthritis—nonsteroidal anti-inflam-

matories and cortisone injections, for example—can have very extreme side effects.

We know now that we can trust this new treatment, not only because of the wealth of clinical research proving that glucosamine and chondroitin sulfates work in both humans and animals, but also because clinical and statistical research in both the United States and Europe reveals the long-standing benefits of this regimen.

As *The Arthritis Cure* showed us, healthy eating is a key component in achieving the best results. Therefore, to unlock the secrets of a healthy, joint-preserving diet, *The Arthritis Cure Cookbook* will introduce seven guidelines to illustrate how you can easily (and deliciously) vary your eating habits to ease the symptoms of osteoarthritis. From this enlightened starting point, you'll be well-equipped to prepare and enjoy the many savory and easy-to-make recipes we've designed especially for you.

About the Recipes in This Book

Many people will find the foods and ideas about cooking and health contained in this book quite new and revolutionary.

For those who already eat a healthy, natural diet, you will certainly find some fresh ideas and new tips. The purpose of this book is to do more than provide you with tasty recipes for healthy eating. We also want to educate you about the healing properties of certain foods, herbs, and spices, and their importance. These recipes have been designed using the foods, spices, and nutrients in quantities that are needed to help preserve healthy joints and encourage the strengthening of damaged ones. If you're cooking for your spouse or family, rest assured that they'll always be glad to see these delicious foods on the table—and you'll be boosting their health and well-being at the same time.

If the ideas and recipes in this book seem like too radical a change from the way you currently eat, try making one change at a time. Substitute your supermarket cereal with a high-fiber, low-sugar one. Consider replacing your morning bagel and cream cheese with whole grain bread, almond butter, and all-fruit conserves, or start using extra virgin olive oil in place of more highly processed ones. You'll notice how your palate will slowly become accustomed to these new tastes as the richness of food's natural flavor emerges. Even small changes in your diet can increase your desire for fresh whole foods, and their healing properties will begin to produce healthy results.

The recipes we've created offer a wide range of flavors. They use ingredients that you're already familiar with, and introduce many new, international ones too. You'll notice how we season with spices such as ginger, cinnamon, cardamom, and garlic. Studies have shown that these spices have natural anti-inflammatory properties. In addition, we've steered away from elaborate recipes, or those that call for a lot of chopping or grinding, since they can be challenging to strained muscles and joints.

We also suggest a wide variety of foods. Maybe the best guideline to follow when preparing meals is what we call the "rainbow plan." If your plate contains a bounty of colorful foods—brown rice, orange carrots or squash, and beautiful greens—then chances are you're eating right. Foods like these, in all their natural glory, have wide ranges of flavor. They don't need artificial additives or extra fat to taste good. The simple addition of herbs and spices can transform a simple vegetable dish into a culinary delight.

Rich-tasting ingredients that you may have eliminated from your diet, such as butter and cream, are used in small amounts in many of the recipes here. Some foods that you may have steered away from in the past, such as eggs, nuts, and even red meat, are also found in some selections. We believe that these foods have a place in your diet because of their nutritional makeup, and again, strongly encourage you to understand how eating a variety of foods in moderation will not only make your meals more enjoyable, but will also be beneficial to your health.

Because everyone chooses a different lifestyle, we've made sure that there are plenty of appetizing and healthful foods to prepare, whatever your personal preferences. You'll find menus that are completely vegetarian and ones that include animal products. We also explain the healthful values of each recipe, which in turn will help you better understand "why" and "how" certain foods work to boost your body's natural defenses.

We steer you away from processed foods not only because they often lack the important nutrients that you need to stay healthy, but because they can often include additives that can make your condition worse. Unfortunately, processed foods are the most common items in the supermarket—but steering clear of them is easy once you know how to read labels and look for other options. But again, don't try to make all your transitions at once. Start by adding a food that is more nutrient-dense and eliminate one that is highly processed and full of additives.

We also want to stress the fact that healthy eating, in and of itself, is not a cure for arthritis. Certainly statistics have increasingly indicated that a healthy diet, combined with the other elements of *The Arthritis Cure*, will help reduce the symptoms of osteoarthritis. However, you may find that diet alone does not offer the significant improvement you desire. But do remember that while dietary changes can positively affect some people in a short period of time, for many others positive results take time. It may be several months before you notice improvement. In the meantime, positive dietary choices can help to maintain your overall health.

As you'll see, the guidelines contained in this book contain information on healthy cooking and, in many cases, "Healthful Hints" on how certain ingredients in the recipe work for you. Preparation and cooking time icons tell you how long a dish will take to prepare so you can better plan your day.

So, try a few of these recipes out. You'll find that by applying the principles of healthy eating and the cooking tips contained in this book, you'll feel better and will enjoy increased energy and vitality.

Bon Appetit!

Seven Guidelines to a Healthful, Joint-Preserving Diet

The types of dietary changes that you make in following *The Arthritis Cure* need not be limiting or difficult to live with—although you may experience some challenges while modifying your usual routine. Remember: Anything new takes some adjustment, and eating better means living a better life.

Before making any type of health care commitment, you and your doctor should determine how much you need to change your diet. But even small changes will be a step in the right direction. Even if you're one of the many Americans who was raised on the standard meat-and-potatoes diet, you'll be pleasantly surprised at how easy and enjoyable our plan for healthy eating is.

A sense of balance is very important when evaluating your diet. Adherence to a too-strict regimen can prove to be stressful and counterproductive. If the majority of your meals are comprised of healthful foods, then an occasional hamburger or piece of candy won't hurt. But when too few "good" foods are consumed, the body doesn't have a foundation for health.

If you love to cook, you'll find great adventure in our suggestions. Perhaps you see cooking as a necessary evil. If so, there's

something for you to learn as well. Whether you cook every meal from scratch, or put together an occasional meal when you're not going out or ordering in, the seven basic tenets of our plan will make you a more enlightened, better prepared chef and consumer.

Following are the basic guidelines to a healthful, joint-preserving diet. We've tried to state the basic concepts in seven, easy-to-understand components to help you better grasp the connection between healthy eating and relief from arthritis.

These seven components combine to help you create better health, just as the many systems of your body combine to function as a whole. More than just a diet, these guidelines (which have been established through research and clinical studies) will not only help alleviate the symptoms of osteoarthritis, but will also assist you in creating a personal foundation for good health.

1. Eat a whole foods diet:

No matter what your school of thought, health care professionals are increasingly recommending that Americans consume less fat, animal protein, and processed foods; and eat more complex carbohydrates, fruits, and vegetables.

A whole foods diet is a varied diet, filled with different colored vegetables, fruits, and grains; raw seeds and nuts; beans; and fermented milk products such as yogurt. It also incoporates fish, poultry, and soy products like tofu. Ideally, your diet should be lower in animal meats, fats, and cheeses, and higher in low-fat milk products.

Whole foods are foods in their natural state, unprocessed and unrefined. We're talking about complete, natural foods — those that contain all the beneficial nutrients that have been discovered and some that have not yet been discovered. It's the difference between eating a whole orange that still has its bioflavonoids in the pith and membranes, and drinking a glass of pasteurized orange juice which is high only in vitamin C. This is not to say that the glass of orange juice isn't beneficial; it is. However, by making simple adjustments to your diet, you can increase your natural nutrient intake many times over.

Whole grains are far superior to refined grains. When flour is refined, for example, more than twenty nutrients are all but removed. When it is then "enriched," only five or so are added back. Refined white wheat flour is low in nutrients such as vitamin E, copper, manganese, and zinc, to name a few. Some of these are needed for bone health, others to counteract the effects

of arthritis medications. In this book, you will see frequent mentions of whole grains in the recipes because these are the best possible sources of some nutrients. But we understand that changes may be hard to make all at once, so feel free to substitute a less "whole" counterpart on occasion. Our aim is to reduce your aches and pains, not to introduce new ones.

Refined white sugar is another example of a food that should ideally be eliminated in a whole foods diet. Its consumption depletes your body of essential vitamins and minerals. This type of sugar is considered a "stressor" food because it adds additional stresses to your body yet provides it with no benefit. Refined white sugar has no fiber and no nutritive value. This sweetener comes with plenty of empty calories, can lead to excess food intake, and contributes to weight gain. Eating refined white sugar is a poor food choice, and you will not find any in these pages. There are many sweet and delicious recipes you can make without using this harmful sweetener. Yet again, while white sugar does not contribute to good health, a healthy individual can eat it in moderation without compromising their diet as a whole.

These are some of the comparisons between a processed diet and a whole foods diet. The overriding purpose of a whole foods diet is to increase your intake of natural fibers and nutrients, and reduce your intake of fat and sugar. Additionally, studies have shown that people who eat a whole foods diet experience more enjoyment from their meals and are satisfied more quickly. This results in less overeating, making it easier to maintain your health and weight.

2. Eat a variety of foods:

When you eat a wide range of foods you give yourself the benefit of a myriad of nutrients. The standard American diet focuses on a narrow range of food choices: wheat as the grain, beef and chicken for protein, iceberg lettuce and tomatoes for vegetables. And while you may think you're getting a variety of foods in one day; if you're eating eggs, bacon, and hash browns for breakfast, it's the same nutritionally as a lunch of a hamburger and French fries or a dinner of a steak and baked potato. While these foods are fine—and even delicious—to eat in moderation,

eaten routinely they limit our nutrient intake. Studies are also revealing that daily consumption of refined, processed foods can lead to a hypersensitivity toward these foods, making our bodies more susceptible to heartburn, gas, and indigestion, among other discomforts.

Our ancestors consumed a variety of foods by eating fruits and vegetables that seasonally came from the earth, and supplemented those with meat. As a result, different seasons yielded different foods and diets varied dramatically. You can vary your own diet according to the season by shopping at local farmers' markets, where the produce comes directly from the growers. Also, look for lower-priced seasonal fruits and vegetables at your supermarket. You can eat well and save money too.

Experiment with spices, seasonings, and different foods. Many people like to experiment with exotic cuisines such as Indian, Chinese, Thai, Japanese, Mexican, African,

Stocking the Shelves

One easy way to ensure that you have the right kinds of foods when you need them is to shop ahead of time. When you're hungry, you don't want to have to run to the grocery store or even worse, the nearest fast food stand. By filling your shelves with healthy, whole food products before you need them, you can increase the likelihood that you'll use them when it's time to prepare a meal.

or Middle Eastern, to name a few. Not only do these foods provide variety, many of the seasonings traditionally used in ethnic cooking have healing properties. Look for a variety of exotic recipes throughout the book, including Mediterranean Cucumber Tzatziki (page 48), Singapore-Style Chicken with Satay Sauce (page 124), and Hindi Ginger Cookies (page 177).

Think of your plate as a painter's palette. Look for the brilliant reds, greens, yellows, and oranges of nature, not the browns and beiges of the major manufacturers. This is an easy way to get a broad sampling of nutrients without having to calculate the nutritional composition of every food. Remember, cooking and eating a healthy diet can be a joy—once you know the secrets.

3. Focus on foods that reduce inflammation:

When there is tissue damage or over-use of a diseased joint as in arthritis, the body's natural response is to send white blood cells to the affected area, causing inflammation. These cells produce prostaglandins and leukotrienes which in turn create a multitude of biochemical reactions. These are meant to heal the area, but also cause joints to feel stiff, warm, swollen, and achy.

Fortunately, nature always provides a remedy. Certain fatty acids in foods are known to counteract the inflammation response.

Alpha-linolenic acid (ALA) is found in green vegetables and other plant foods. This is an omega-3 fatty acid that blocks the specific kinds of prostaglandins and leukotrienes that cause inflammation.

Eicosapentaenoic acid (EPA) is found in marine plants and fish, especially fatty fish such as salmon and sardines. If you can, try to eat fish twice a week—more if possible. If possible, poach or broil fish because frying adds fat and destroys omega-3's.

Linoleic acid is found in corn, soybean, and other plant oils and is a precursor to EPA. It cannot be synthesized from other nutrients, but allows your body to make other fatty acids.

Gamma-linolenic acid (GLA) can be taken as a supplement, in black currant oil, evening primrose oil, and borage seed oil. These are also precursors to the kinds of prostaglandins that reduce inflammation.

"Trans-fatty acids" is a buzzword being circulated today that bears a lot of weight but has little meaning for most Americans. Simply put, a trans-fatty acid is a man-made molecule which may interfere with normal metabolic functions because their unusual molecular shape isn't readily recognized by our systems. Our cell membranes, our immune systems, and our overall ability to heal are then compromised because an "outsider" has been introduced to the body; one that forces us to change to its rules, rather than one that adapts to our natural chemistry. Rather than contributing to the body's miraculous functions, trans-fatty acids are actually destroying them.

Trans-fatty acids can be identified on food labels which use "partially hydrogenated oil" as an ingredient. Many processed food products contain these hydrogenated oils, and the United States has recently insisted that all package labeling must measure and identify the types of fat in every product. To easily avoid these products, choose butter over margarine; olive and flaxseed oils over the many processed oils available; fresh vegetables over canned and processed ones; and make reading labels a part of your shopping routine.

4. Choose foods that contain antioxidants:

One leading theory of what causes us to age is the free-radical theory. Free radicals are unstable molecules that roam about the body, attacking and destroying healthy tissue, including the tissue found in the joints.

Good oils versus bad oils

When oils are overheated and used for too long, such as in fast food restaurants, they become oxidized. Oxidized oils are loaded with oxygen-damaging free radicals (cell-destroying molecules). To counteract the dangers of free radicals, many doctors suggest supplementing your diet with vitamin and mineral supplements. You can protect your metabolic processes and cell membranes with antioxidants such as vitamins C, A (or beta-carotene), and E, plus the mineral antioxidant selenium. Optimally, you would get these vitamins and minerals through diet and higher doses (in the form of supplementation) are often required to fend off the dangerous by-products of chemically processed foods.

When choosing an oil to cook with, think natural. Olive and flaxseed oils are far superior to processed oils, and butter is better than margarine.

It's also better to cook with vegetable oils only at low temperatures. (And if you increase your "bad oil" intake, also remember to increase your antioxidants!)

Osteoarthritis may be the result of free radical damage, and joint inflammation itself may trigger an even faster rate of new free radical formation.

Fortunately there is an antidote for free radicals: antioxidants that join with these unstable molecules and stabilize them, preventing them from doing more harm. Antioxidants are not at all new, just the old familiar vitamin A (beta-carotene and the other carotenoids which are the plant form of the vitamin), vitamin C, and vitamin E, plus the mineral selenium.

Where are these antioxidants found? Most often in the fruits and vegetables that make up a whole foods diet.

Vitamin A and the carotenoids: Vitamin A is necessary for healthy cell growth, and is commonly considered the vitamin that gives you lustrous hair, clear skin, and good vision.

While vitamin A itself is found in animal foods such as liver and eggs, its precursor, beta-carotene, and the other carotenoids are found in plant foods. Beta-carotene also happens to be the pigment orange, so look for orange-colored fruits and vegetables when you shop for dinner and you can be sure you are including this antioxidant in your meals.

Vitamin C: This antioxidant is in many fruits and vegetables besides oranges. Bell peppers have higher amounts per calorie than citrus, although the many varieties of citrus make vitamin C a relatively easy nutrient to get. Cabbage (any color) is also an excellent form of this essential antioxidant, and its vitamins are shared whether the cabbage is raw or cooked.

Vitamin E: An essential antioxidant which protects red blood cells and is essential in keeping cell walls flexible and healthy, vitamin E is a nutrient lacking in most diets.

This fat-soluble vitamin is in short supply in the American diet because it's contained in the germ of the grain that is removed when refining whole grain flours into white flour. It's also missing in processed oils. For good health, eat whole grains and unprocessed oils. Asparagus and spinach are two excellent, delicious, natural forms of vitamin E.

Selenium: This mineral is considered the active partner of vitamin E, helping the body to utilize it. You can find it in sunflower seeds, swordfish, salmon, and shrimp.

A good way to increase your antioxidant intake is through juicing. See step 7 for more information on the nutritional benefits of juicing. Recipes for delicious nutrient-filled smoothies begin on page 183.

5. Include foods high in bioflavonoids:

Found in virtually all plant foods, bioflavonoids are essential in helping the body regenerate itself in a healthy way. They are essential for maintaining healthy capillary walls and metabolizing vitamin C, needed for building connective tissue. If you suffer from osteoarthritis, bioflavonoids can also be helpful by supporting your body's ability to manufacture collagen for the delicate connective tissue between your joints. Other important uses are:

- Preventing cellular damage from free radicals;
- Slowing the body's natural inflammation response;
- Preventing collagen destruction when the cartilage tissue is inflamed; and
- Speeding up the healing process of an injury.

Citrus is an excellent source of bioflavonoids, and is found in the pith and membranes of the fruit and in the central core. You enjoy the healthiest benefits of an orange when you eat it by the slice. Other excellent foods are green tea, berries, onions, and all fruits that contain a pit.

Bioflavonoids are also found in buckwheat (sometimes referred to as kasha). Instead of having a standard wheat dinner roll with your meal, cook some kasha,

News You Can Use on Arthritis

The latest clinical research suggests that certain vitamins, minerals and nutrients are the most effective way of augmenting the effectiveness of glucosamine and chondroitin sulfates, as referenced in *The Arthritis Cure*. The following daily minimum amounts are recommended*:

Vitamin A	5000 IU
Vitamin C	500 mg
Vitamin E	150 IU
Calcium	300 mg
Magnesium	100 mg
Copper	1 mg
Zinc	5 mg
Boron	1.5 mg
Chromium	50 mcg
Selenium	50 mcg
Manganese	10 mg
Silicon	5 mg

*They are discussed in detail in *Maximizing the Arthritis Cure* (St. Martin's Press, available in bookstores or by calling 1-800-321-9299).

Russian style, with onions and mushrooms or try some Japanese soba noodles (also made from buckwheat) in a soup or a side dish.

6. Maintain your ideal body weight:

Let's be very clear that "ideal body weight" is not the same as the weight of movie stars and fashion models. Ideal body weight is the size and amount that is most comfortable and appropriate for your body. Keep in mind that there are many variables to weight depending on frame size and muscle tone.

If you believe that you need to reduce your weight to take pressure off your arthritic joints, you're probably right. So let that be your primary motivational factor. You can't manage your weight for someone else—do it for yourself and your good health.

The first step to remember when losing weight is to eat. This may sound silly, but skipping meals can lower your metabolic rate, thus slowing your body's systems down. This means that not only does your body not have enough fuel to operate properly, it also doesn't have enough energy to burn fat. Also, when you skip a meal or forget to eat, you're more likely to make poor food choices with your next meal.

If you are eating a diet full of nutrients (predominantly from whole, unprocessed, unrefined foods) your body won't have continual cravings for more food. Hunger is sated when your body is truly fed, not when you fill it with empty calories. Eat well, and your ideal body weight will start to reveal itself.

Of course it's important not to binge on fatty foods, but your body will ask for fat. When it does, give it healthy vegetable oils and oily fish products such as salmon. These fats can reduce the inflammation often associated with arthritis and will also satisfy your hunger.

It's also important to stay away from large amounts of sweets. Pouring these molecules of glucose into your system rapidly will trigger your body to store the sugar as fat. Sugar that cannot be stored as ready-energy turns to acid in the system. Your body wants to neutralize that acid quickly, hence the conversion to fat and hard-to-lose pounds.

Don't forget to exercise, even if it's just walking up that flight of stairs to your apartment or office. Exercise increases your metabolic rate and has the added benefit of stimulating the body to build healthy cartilage.

Remember that a weight loss of 1 to 2 pounds a week is the optimal healthy rate of weight loss. Don't be discouraged if your progress isn't that rapid. "Thin Thighs in Ten Days," is a gimmick. A healthy body on the other hand, is an investment of time and energy.

7. Replace nutrients depleted by prescription drugs:

Drugs prescribed for arthritis—primarily nonsteroidal anti-inflammatory drugs (NSAIDs) and other medications—can leech nutrients from the body. If you are taking any of these drugs, you need to pay special attention to your diet and eat foods high in nutrients you may be missing.

For example, many common NSAIDs (including ones sold over-the-counter) decrease levels of vitamin C in the body. Good natural sources of vitamin C are peppers, citrus fruits, and cabbage; whereas carrots provide an excellent source of beta-carotene, an antioxidant.

Juicing is an easy and efficient way to absorb the high levels of nutrients stored in fruits and vegetables. For example, it takes approximately five pounds of carrots to produce one quart of carrot juice. It would be almost impossible to eat five pounds of carrots in one day, but relatively easy to drink a quart of juice.

It's a good idea to have your physician or a qualified nutritionist measure your nutrient levels in the blood and tissue. Have a reading done on your levels of vitamin C, folic acid, phosphorous, zinc, and potassium. And, if recommended, eat foods high in these nutrients.

Another concern that goes in tandem with prescription drugs is the use of

---

Seven Guidelines to a Healthful, Joint-Preserving Diet Recap

1. **Eat a whole foods diet.** Basic, unprocessed, natural foods whenever possible.
2. **Eat a variety of foods.** Remember to eat a rainbow of colors.
3. **Focus on inflammation-reducing foods.** Avoid trans-fatty acids.
4. **Choose foods high in antioxidants.** Attack the free radicals, protect your joints.
5. **Include foods high in bioflavonoids.** Supplement your body with these natural immune boosters.
6. **Maintain your ideal body weight.** Do it for yourself and your health.
7. **Replace nutrients depleted by prescription drugs.** Up your intake of vitamins and minerals by juicing.

antacids containing aluminum or magnesium hydroxide. Often, these are taken to combat the stomach upset of prescription and over-the-counter medications. Yet, they can leech vital phosphorus from your body—one of the minerals necessary to keep your bones strong. You can counter this loss by eating foods high in phosphorus such as lean meats, lowfat milk and yogurt, soybeans, peanut butter, green leafy vegetables, oranges, nuts, and seeds.

These seven guidelines are implemented throughout the book. As you can see, they all work together—much like your body's various systems. In the following chapters, you'll note how each recipe offers nutritional information to help you make the best possible food choices using the basic tenets of *The Arthritis Cure*. We've done our best to make this book as informative and as interesting as possible. Now it's up to you. Cook and eat your way to good health!

The Arthritis-Friendly Kitchen

Cooking even the simplest meal requires considerable dexterity: chop the tomato, get out the colander, drain the pasta, grate the parmesan. In the main section of this book, the recipes have been structured to minimize manual labor, but food preparation still places some demands on joints in wrists, fingers, elbows, and shoulders. Cooking can also be tiring on the legs and feet.

To minimize the strain on your body, here are some tips for the arthritis-friendly kitchen. From the details of proper posture to designing your kitchen to choosing equipment, we've tried to compile information that will help make cooking as easy and enjoyable as possible. The reality is that you're not going to want to cook if it makes you overly tired, so here are some suggestions for maximizing your energy and reintroducing the fun back into your kitchen.

This chapter is divided into four parts. Part One discusses how you can maximize your energy and offers tips for relaxation and rediscovering the joy in cooking. Part Two explores the obstacles you face in the kitchen—from replacing or updating poorly designed cookware to quick, easy, and inexpensive ways to update your kitchen utensils. For those with a passion for cooking (and a budget to match), Part Three offers suggestions on revamping or remodeling your kitchen. And because we consider the mind to be the body's equal partner in the healing process, Part Four addresses the difficult, but necessary task of asking for help and support.

Do yourself a favor and consider these changes now. You'll be surprised at what a new philosophy and a few kitchen secrets will bring to your experience.

PART ONE:
There's happiness in cooking

For some of you, the possibility of being inspired in the kitchen may seem pretty remote. But there are ways to get cooking again if you take steps to combat the pain and fatigue that have been literally "cramping your style".

As you well know, cooking involves more than simply preparing a meal. It means planning, shopping, preparing, cooking, and cleaning up. No wonder the thought of it can make you tired. Still, changing or modifying some of your daily habits can relieve the stress on your mind and body. Try out a few of the following:

Steps to relieve stress and fatigue

Think of ways to reduce fatigue and minimize stress to fragile joints. Being aware of the challenges you face in the kitchen is the first step to jumping back into cooking.

Try to work from a sitting position

While this may seem unnatural at first, sitting down offers an opportunity to support your body. Remember to keep your feet on the floor and your back supported by a good, straight-backed chair. Let the table support your upper arms by resting your elbows on the table, and use your forearms for the actual work.

Be sure that your work surface is the correct height

Whether sitting or standing, your work surface should fall just a bit below your elbow level. If you have to bend over, you're working too hard.

Be aware of your level of fatigue

If you get too tired, stop and take a break. Try combining several tasks at once to conserve your energy and get the most out of your efforts. Start by preparing recipes that can be interrupted if you need to take a break.

Try to minimize lifting

Lifting takes a lot of energy and can easily wear you out. Try to brainstorm ideas that will help you reduce your lifting, such as using a wire basket to cook vegetables (so you don't have to drain the heavy pan in the sink), or by keeping recipe ingredients close at hand.

Wear good shoes

If you're going to be on your feet, wear good shoes. Consider buying a pair with added arch support and extra cushioning. You don't need to use them only for cooking; wear them for any activity that involves a lot of standing or walking.

Use some of the labor-saving gadgets discussed in Part Two

Though some of these products may seem hard to get used to, over time they'll make the job so much easier. Don't try to

---

5 Habits to Keep Your Energy Level Up

1. Rest before you get tired.
2. Alternate easy and difficult household tasks.
3. Organize your workspace.
4. Shop for pre-cut or pre-packaged foods.
5. Use labor-saving devices such as a blender, electric can opener, or food processor.

lift a heavy skillet by the handle alone. It can add a great deal of strain to your hands and arms. Instead, look into purchasing skillet "clip-on" handles that allow you to disperse the weight evenly between your arms and hands—without getting burned.

Learning to enjoy cooking again

Your minutes or hours spent in the kitchen need not be boring. Sure, you may have been turning out meals for your family for years, but a new understanding about how food affects your health and well-being can give you the jump-start you need to begin cooking with newfound interest and creativity. Here are some shopping strategies:

Shop someplace new. Does your town have farmers' or open-air markets? Many communities today host local farmers once or twice a week. Here you'll find the freshest produce, exotic Asian vegetables, bouquets of spinach, and oddities such as brussels sprouts still on the stalk. Many markets also feature fresh-baked breads, nuts, dried fruit, fresh fish, meat, eggs, and plants or flowers.

There's also a healthy bonus to shopping

10 Quick Tips for the Arthritis-Friendly Kitchen

1. Wear an apron with pockets. Carry the objects or tools you use most frequently in your pockets so they'll be handy when you need them.

2. Keep a pair of kitchen scissors handy. They can be used for everything from cutting open cellophane bags to trimming lettuce and parsley.

3. Use your sink's sprayer hose to fill pots with water. Fill the pots on the counter so you don't have to lift a heavy pot out of the sink.

4. Cook vegetables and pasta in a pot lined with a mesh basket. When you lift up the basket, the water will automatically drain out.

5. Attach a brush with suction cups to the inside of your sink for scrubbing vegetables.

6. Add suction cups to the bottom of your cutting board so it doesn't move around.

7. Use lightweight, plastic mixing bowls.

8. Use lightweight utensils and plates whenever possible.

9. Press out the moisture in a damp cloth rather than wringing it dry.

10. Take breaks.

this way. Because the produce is always of the season and fresh-picked, you can trust that the nutrient content is high in what you buy. Certain nutrients will develop only when a vegetable is ripened in the field, not picked early to ripen en route to the supermarket.

If you're lucky enough to have a farmers' market in your area, go and let the produce inspire your next meal. Be forewarned, you'll probably buy more than you can carry so it's a good idea to pack a lightweight folding cart to help you get the goods home.

Ethnic food shops can be very entertaining, and you'll find them in just about every town or city today. Be adventurous and visit that aromatic, cluttered little Indian market you've passed so many times. You'll find fresh spices of every description, nuts, herbs, and exotic condiments.

Make a special effort to shop at the Italian deli where you can buy chunks of Romano cheese that they'll grate for you. It's much tastier than the pre-packaged cheeses you'll find in the supermarket. Visit a Spanish or Greek market for all kinds of dried beans, and be sure to pick up some extra virgin olive oil, too.

When you go to your usual supermarket, meander down aisles you normally skip. Many stores now have ethnic food shelves, catering to changing tastes. In addition to your staples, you may also come home with something wonderful, different, and joint-enhancing to try.

Visit a natural foods supermarket too. There are now several chains that have opened across America that feature relatively unprocessed, unrefined whole foods, the kind that used to be only in health food stores. Here you'll find a much wider variety of whole grains, breakfast cereals, baked goods, cheeses, prepared foods, and produce than the larger supermarkets.

For those who are more homebound, check out our list of mail order sources in the back of the book. Most of these merchants have catalogs and 800 numbers for your convenience, and you can enjoy the finest ingredients delivered right to your door.

Cook with new ingredients. Never in human history has such an array of foods been so widely available. All the foods of the world's cuisine pour into our markets in the United States. There are chili condiments from Thailand and perfumed fruits such as cherimoyas from the Caribbean. Ever since the kiwi hit our shores, gourmet food importers have been looking for more exotics to bring to our table. There's also a wider range of home-grown produce in the stores. Greens such as collards, chard, and kale used in Southern cooking are now regularly found in supermarkets throughout the states.

Many of these new-to-us foods are time-honored classic ingredients of international cuisine. These same foods have supported life for thousands of years, and many cultures have acknowledged their medicinal uses and health benefits, including the treatment of arthritis. Many of the recipes here include spices that reduce inflammation, orange vegetables high in antioxidants, and healthful fish and nuts with the same beneficial oils that have kept traditional peoples arthritis-free for generations.

Try a new recipe or rethink some of your old ones, using healthful ingredients. Make some homemade pizza using whole-wheat English muffin halves with sliced vegetables and some of your own sauce. Or easier yet, take a slice of Italian bread and toast it. Rub the toast with a clove of garlic (the toasted bread will act like a grater), drizzle with olive oil, and top it with a slice or two of ruby red tomato and sprinkle with grated cheese. Eat as is or broil and enjoy!

Remember, you don't have to follow a recipe exactly. Use it as a jumping off place, and invent as you go. Think of cooking as a chance to use your talents, be creative, and indulge your whims.

Care for the Cook. Feed yourself while you cook to keep your energy flowing, reduce strain on joints, and quiet your hunger. Have a tall glass of fruit juice mixed with water (half and half), to keep from wilting. Take a few deep breaths, straighten out your spine, and stretch your arms and shoulders to relax them. Stand on your toes for a second to stretch your feet and calf muscles.

Spice up your environment by putting a few of your favorite things in the kitchen — maybe it's a family picture, a vase with fresh flowers, or a special memento. Turn on some music. Many people find cooking to be a peaceful interval which is very nurturing.

Double-Cook. Leave more time for the fun part — eating! Use a crock-pot and have your dinner cook itself all day long. Roast a chicken for tomorrow while you eat dinner tonight.

Leftovers too, can be the basis for many new dishes. Our Mexican Succotash (page 102) changes into a soup just by adding water and a little salt and pepper. The Yucatan Citrus Black Bean Soup (page 87) becomes a filling for corn tortillas — just cook out the liquid in a wide frying pan and add a little chili powder. Grilled Swordfish with Mango-Papaya Salsa (page 134) is the beginning of a fish salad served with whole wheat pita bread. Bring a bit of your own creativity to the kitchen, and there is no end to the delicious food you can create.

PART TWO:
Treat yourself to some new cooking tools

As you begin cooking again you'll enjoy it more if you allow yourself to be tempted by those incredible housewares stores. Give yourself permission to buy an ice cream maker (there are some today that won't break the bank). You can make colorful, healthful sorbets that fit right into your new eating plan. Or you may find some beautifully engineered measuring cups, or a very fine paring or garnishing knife that will bring a certain finesse to your food presentation. There is pleasure in finding the right tools for the right task.

At the very least, take inventory of the utensils you have and see if anything needs to be replaced. There is no point in working harder than you need to. Do your knives need sharpening? Have you "made do" with a measuring cup with the numbers worn off? If so, treat yourself to some new items. After all, if you're not going to take care of yourself, who is?

Remember when reviewing the following list, it's not necessary to run out and buy everything at once. You may find that you don't want—or even need—some of them. Consider the kitchen tasks you perform most often and those that give you the most pain or difficulty. Then purchase one or two of the kitchen tools that promise to remedy your situation and give them a try.

What to look for in a kitchen tool:

In choosing appliances, utensils, and kitchen hardware, look for items that favor the use of the arm rather than the hand. Think of your hand as another utensil, while your real strength is in the arm. You don't want to buy products that will require a twisting action in your wrist in order to use them. Look for designs that require just a little push, a pressing action, or products that allow you to use both hands at once. Invest in a garlic press, a portable chopper, or a spice grinder. Always use electricity to your advantage—an electric can opener or mixer is easier on your wrists than a manual one.

Labor-saving kitchen appliances:

Blenders and Juicers: Everyone has a blender stored somewhere in the house. Get it out and start pureeing. They're great for making soups, sauces, and frothy drinks, and can be used as a vegetable chopper, using the pulse button. (See page 183 for delicious recipes that you can make in your blender.)

Juicers take a little more manual dexterity to use, but are worth the extra effort. When fruits and vegetables are juiced, nutrients are more readily absorbed by the body. If you are trying to boost your antioxidant intake, think juice.

Choppers: We all know the larger food processors that have become a staple in modern kitchens, but don't forget about the small versions. While you may not have the need for a full sized processor, when you need to chop half an onion or mince a few sprigs of parsley, you'll be glad to have a smaller version in your kitchen.

Some models have about a 1½ cup capacity, and their rotary blade can chop vegetables, herbs, nuts, cheese, and meat as well as blend homemade mayonnaise and sauces. They operate with a touch of a button and have easy-grip lids.

There are also electric cheese grinders for the cheese lover, nutmeg grinders for the baker, and electric pepper mills for wonderful fresh-ground pepper. If you love pepper, you may want two—one for white peppercorns, one for black.

Crock Pot: These electric cookers can simplify cooking in a big way. Put your grains, beans, vegetables, and herbs on in the morning, slow cook all day, and return at night to a nicely cooked soup or stew. One-pot meals cut down on kitchen work and make for healthy leftovers.

Electric Mixer: This is another classic. Electric mixers are inexpensive to buy, and when a recipe reads "mix," "whip," or "beat," you can, and with little effort. The newer models also have the advantage of being much lighter than the older ones.

Smart Cookware: Buy pots and pans that are light-weight and well-balanced. Quality pots cook evenly and burn less often. You'll save time on washing as well. For health reasons, use pots without an aluminum interior. Look for pots with handles that curve downward. Because of the leverage involved, these are easiest to lift. Again, you don't have to run out and buy a whole new set if you don't need one. See if any of your current cookware needs replacing, and try out a new style one pan at a time.

Utensils to make the job easier:

It would be virtually impossible to list every available kitchen tool or gadget, but these are the ones that really help make life easier. Some of the following utensils may already be in your kitchen drawer. If not, you may find that they are worth adding to your collection.

Adjustable Pot Clamp: These vinyl-cushioned long handles clamp on to the rim of your existing pots, one on each side, to help you lift a heavy load. They are adjustable—and indispensable.

Ceramic Utensil Pot: A useful accessory in a French country kitchen is a homey ceramic pot, about 6 inches wide and 10 or 12 inches deep. It's meant to hold regularly used kitchen utensils—the wooden spoon, the spatula, the slotted spoon. And keeping utensils in easy reach is easier on you.

Garlic Peeler: A floppy plastic tube doesn't look like the greatest garlic peeler ever, but it is! Insert whole, unpeeled cloves in the tube, press down firmly, and briskly roll back and forth for a few seconds until you hear the garlic peel snap. The peeled cloves roll right out, and the skins stick to the inside until rinsed away in the sink.

Hands-free Waste Bin: Invest in a new waste bin that you tap on a pedal to open.

There is also one that stays open and then closes with another tap.

Jar Opener Aids: There are a variety of these to try. One, the "jar key," provides leverage for opening jars by popping the vacuum seal. Another provides extra grip for twisting off caps and lids. A "jar vise" mounts under the shelf to help do the same thing. Use both hands to turn the jar.

Knives: Buy good quality ones and keep them sharp. The sharper the knife, the less effort from you. Take your knives to a professional knife sharpener once a year, and then use a diamond dust sharpening tool to maintain the new edge.

Mezzaluna: This is a most useful cutting implement. It means 'half-moon' in Italian, referring to its curved shape. With a handle at each end, it's perfect for a person with arthritis. With a mezzaluna, food can be chopped, or pizza sliced with a rocking motion.

Storage Containers: When you need to store cooked food, use plastic or glass containers with flexible lids, rather than containers with screw-on tops. They seal with a gentle press.

Utensils with Rubber Grip Handles: Rubber grips promote a firm grip and are easy to hold. Whisks, potato peelers, ladles, and the like are fitted with rubber for secure and easy handling.

Whisk: The multiple loops of heavy wire that join to form a whisk produce more mixing per stroke than stirring with a spoon or fork. The French knew what they were doing when they invented this. Look for one with a wide rubber handle.

The various items you need to adapt your kitchen can be found in housewares stores, hardware stores, and gourmet shops. These days, it seems that even the supermarket is getting into the game. Also, keep an eye on your mail—catalogues for these products are likely to show up on your doorstep.

PART THREE:
Revamping your kitchen

If you need to adapt your kitchen to your physical needs, it may suffice to just make a little change in hardware, or it may be necessary to do quite a bit more. The good news is that most existing kitchens can be retrofitted to serve those with arthritis. Here are some suggestions:

Smaller changes

The following are changes that can be made easily and/or inexpensively.

A place to store ingredients out in the open. Get used to the idea that it's more convenient to store commonly used ingredients out in the open—where they're easy to get to. Clear off a shelf or have one installed in your cooking area for spices, herbs, and frequently used foods. It will cut down on the labor of toting ingredients back and forth.

A large table, designed for food prepara-
tion. As we mentioned in Part One, it's
much easier on the body to prepare food
while sitting down at a table. Look for a
large table that is the proper height for
your needs and make room for it in your
kitchen. If you're undergoing a full-scale
remodeling, consider integrating a table
into your design.

Extend handles on doors and water
faucets. These longer handles can be easily
acquired at a good hardware store or home
design center. By extending the handles,
you can easily take advantage of extended
leverage to open doors and turn water on
and off.

Look for lever handles on cabinets.
Changing the handles on your cabinets can
save a lot of extra wrist and elbow work in
pulling and pressing. An easy press downward, and the door opens. Conversely, you
can nudge the door back in place and the
level will latch the cabinet again.

Buy some hooks, and hang your aprons,
dish towels, and cooking mitts where you can
reach them effortlessly. It may seem obvi-
ous, but too many cooks stash their cooking mitts in drawers. That means bending
over and rummaging through drawers
when you need something. Keep these vital
items handy and you'll be surprised how
every little movement you save helps
increase your stamina in the kitchen.

Larger changes

You might want to factor in the suggestions below if you are considering remodeling or major reworking of your kitchen
work space.

- Consider a country look for your shelves
  and pantry. Store dishware and staples
  on open shelves. Remove cabinet doors
  or install new shelving. Put everything
  within easy reach. Foods such as pasta,
  rice, and flour can be very attractive
  stored in clear containers.
- Install flooring with some flexibility.
  Today, floors can be laid with material
  that makes walking and standing less of
  a chore on the back, neck, and spine.
- Plastic-coated wire shelving. For storing
  cookware, plastic coated shelving is
  ideal. Hang pots from hooks on the
  shelving or on a pot rack for good looks
  and great function. Always install pot
  shelves close to your workspace or range
  at a level you can easily reach. Your
  cookware will be organized, out of the
  way, and yet handy.

Rolling trolleys. If you decide you like
the look of kitchenware behind closed
doors, at least mount your shelves on good
quality rolling trolleys so that they easily
roll out to give you easy access to what is
stored in the rear and corners.

Good lighting. Seeing exactly what
you're doing is crucial. Hire a knowledge-
able electrician or consult with a designer

(a student in a design school would love the assignment and could probably use it for course credit) and have them work out a lighting plan. Good general lighting as well as task lighting is a real plus. Or install lighting under suspended cabinets to illuminate a counter working space.

PART FOUR:
Asking for support

Smart self-sufficiency means knowing when to ask for help. No one can do everything alone, and if you begin to view your limitations as obstacles to be hurdled — rather than as barriers to full participation — you'll have the right mindset to put you on the road to recovery. Here are a few generalized suggestions:

Most supermarkets, and all butcher and fish shops, will clean and debone meats and fish and will slice them to your specifications with a minimum purchase. Some may charge a nominal fee. Take advantage of this benefit when possible.

Many forms of salad greens can be purchased already washed and stemmed, in pre-packaged bags. Try flavorful baby greens and spinach — which can be steamed with a bit of olive oil for a quick, healthy side dish.

Cabbage, carrots, broccoli, and other crunchy vegetables are commonly sold in pre-washed, pre-chopped forms. Some markets even offer a "vegetable medley" of pre-cut seasonal vegetables. They are perfect for a quick stir-fry with some Japanese soba (buckwheat) noodles.

Many large supermarkets and specialty grocers offer telephone shopping and delivery services. Often, these services are free or discounted if you purchase a certain dollar amount. And if you're eligible, don't pass up those senior citizen discounts, either.

Barter with another great cook. If you're fortunate enough to know another great cook in your community, propose a barter system with that person or family. They can provide one (or two) full meals a week while you provide the same number in exchange. They may be a superb baker, and you prefer cooking soups and stews. Just cook twice as much and pass it on! Not only do you get to sample someone else's good cooking, but you get to take some time off from the kitchen!

Create a cooking party. There are frontstage cooks and backstage cooks. Backstage cooks keep all the preparation secret and perform all the work themselves. Frontstage cooks show it all and can share the effort and the fun. If you have no one to cook for, invite someone over. It can be much more interesting cooking for someone besides yourself, the company is nice, and your guest will probably help out. Make the preparation the focus of the party.

Experiment with the following recipes and turn cooking into a new experience. While cooking is a daily task, it can be a creative outlet, too. Most importantly, begin thinking of your kitchen as a pain-free place to prepare delicious foods that can help heal your arthritis.

 TIME: Indicates how long it will take to prepare and cook each receipe.

 STASH AND SNACK: The dish stores well and can be served later as a snack or side dish.

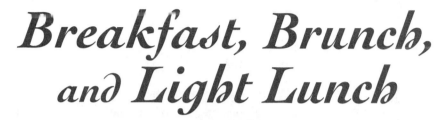

Breakfast, Brunch, and Light Lunch

Easy and Fast Morning Meals, and Light Lunch Suggestions
Old-Fashioned Oatmeal with Sunflower Seeds
Helene's Great Granola
Sunday Morning French Toast with Whipped Strawberry Sauce
Aunt Priscilla's Apricot-Barley Cereal with Grilled Apples
Blueberry Pancakes with Creamy Fruit Topping
Spicy Turkey Patties on English Muffins
Frittata and Omelette Primer with Toppings and Fillings
Russian Sunflower-Rye Muffins
Coconut-Orange Muffins with Walnuts
Southwestern Corn Bread
Shrimp and Swiss Chard Scramble with Pineapple Garnish
South of France Chicken and Olive Sandwiches
Avocado and Watercress Pita with Garlic-Onion Jam
Open-faced Tuna Steak Sandwiches with Sun-dried Tomato Mayonnaise

Easy and Fast Morning Meals and Light Lunch Suggestions

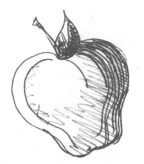

Breakfast

Although we've all heard that breakfast is the most important meal of the day, it is still often one of those meals we consume quickly, grab on the run, or skip altogether. Here are some suggestions for quick, nutritious breakfast foods or light lunches that are great for those on the go!

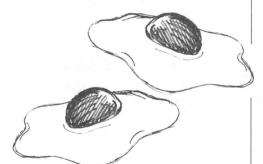

- Whole grain bread, almond butter, and all-fruit conserves.

- Muffins made with whole grain flours and no refined sugars.

- Eggs, in any style (soft or hard boiled, scrambled, or sunny-side up) with sesame whole wheat pita.

- Plain yogurt with active cultures, and sliced fresh fruit or all-fruit conserves.

- Morning cereal favorites from the natural food store such as Brown Rice Crispies, Oatio's, museli, etc., with low salt, no added sugar, fiber intact, and no preservatives. (These are great for snacking, too.)

- Midwestern Cornmeal Wedges (page 57), cooked in some butter, sprinkled with cinnamon, and drizzled with real maple syrup.

Light Lunches

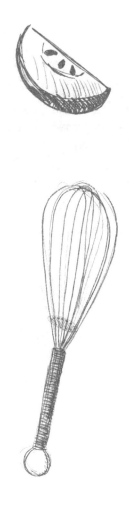

* English muffin (whole grain, of course) and Nutty Mushroom Pâté (see page 47).

* Whole grain toast, a smear of mustard, and tomato slices.

* Open-faced sandwiches with avocado, salad greens, and a slice of tomato with mustard.

* Sardines, red onion rings, and cucumber slices.

* Bowl of bean soup with a hunk of whole grain bread.

* Egg sandwich on a toasted English muffin.

* Any of the lunch suggestions in this chapter.

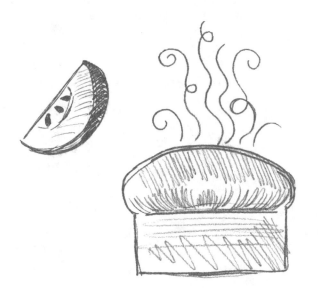

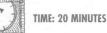

Old-Fashioned Oatmeal with Sunflower Seeds

With the age of instant fully upon us, many haven't tasted the richness of oatmeal from the turn of the century, which contains more of the original nutrients and fiber than its modern counterpart. (If you have a morning time crunch, make a batch on the weekend and reheat a portion each morning.)

2 ½ cups purified water or apple juice

1 cup old-fashioned rolled oats (see Note)

¼ cup raisins or currants, unsulphured preferred

½ teaspoon ground cinnamon

¼ teaspoon sea salt

2 tablespoons real maple syrup

1 tablespoon unsalted butter (optional)

¼ to ½ cup sunflower seeds or walnuts (optional)

Place the water or juice, oatmeal, raisins or currants, cinnamon, and salt in a medium saucepan. Bring to a boil, uncovered, over medium high heat, reduce heat and simmer for 15 minutes, stirring occasionally.

Stir in the maple syrup and butter. If you prefer a thinner consistency, add 2 to 3 tablespoons water or juice.

Add fruit options into the bottom of the bowl, and pour a hearty serving on top. Serve hot. Sprinkle with seeds or nuts to add some EFAs to your day.

YIELD: 4 SERVINGS

HEALTHFUL HINT: If you are accustomed to sweet breakfast cereals, a way to turn up the sweetness, is to mix in one or several of the following fruit options: apple, peach, or banana slices; unsweetened apple butter or sauce; all-fruit conserves.

NOTE: If cooking your oatmeal from scratch seems beyond possibility right now, don't settle for the sugar-laden instant varieties. There are many finely ground whole grain breakfast cereals that cook quickly and are almost instant — and without the added refined sugars!

"All happiness depends on a leisurely breakfast."

—John Gunther

Helene's Great Granola

A family heirloom recipe that's been handed down through the generations, this granola can take on many flavors depending upon which spices, fruit, nuts, and seeds are used. Granola will last several months in the freezer or refrigerator, and it makes a healthy snack.

PREHEAT THE OVEN TO 350 DEGREES.

In a large bowl, combine the rolled oats, walnuts, almonds, sesame seeds, and cinnamon.

In a medium-size saucepan, melt the butter over medium heat. Add the maple syrup, molasses, and salt, and heat until the molasses dissolves. Add the water, apple butter, and vanilla extract and stir again.

Pour the butter mixture into the oatmeal mixture and stir well to coat.

Spread the granola onto two well-buttered baking sheets. Place in the oven. Using a spoon or a spatula, stir the granola every 5 minutes as it bakes. Continue baking until golden brown and crispy, 15 to 20 minutes.

Remove from the oven and pour into a large bowl. Add the dry fruit, toss, and set aside to cool completely. Once cool, store in a covered container in the refrigerator or freezer.

YIELD: 6 CUPS

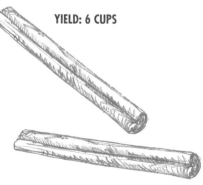

ADDITIONS: Substitute or add coconut, pumpkin seeds, or pecans.

VARIATIONS: Substitute ginger, cardamom, clove, or allspice powder.

NOTE: The granola will be sweeter when made with apple juice.

4 cups old-fashioned rolled oats

½ cup walnuts, coarsely chopped

½ cup almonds, coarsely chopped

½ cup sesame seeds (see Additions)

1 teaspoon cinnamon (see Variations)

¼ cup unsalted butter or ghee

¼ cup real maple syrup or honey

1 tablespoon unsulphured blackstrap molasses

½ teaspoon sea salt

1 cup purified water or unsweetened apple juice (see Note)

½ cup unsweetened apple butter or apple sauce

½ teaspoon real vanilla, almond, lemon, or orange extracts

1 to 2 cups unsweetened dry fruit such as raisins, currants, blueberries, or chopped apricots, apples, or prunes, unsulphured preferred

Sunday Morning French Toast with Whipped Strawberry Sauce

Now you can make wonderful-for-you and delicious French toast with a fancy topping right in your own kitchen. Start out your weekend with this wonderful treat.

2 eggs, organic preferred

1 cup plain yogurt with active cultures

½ cup unsweetened apple juice

4 to 6 slices whole grain bread

2 to 3 tablespoons unsalted butter

Cinnamon

1 recipe Strawberry Sauce (see page 169)

In a blender or food processor, beat the eggs, yogurt, and apple juice.

Pour mixture into a deep 9- x 13-inch rectangular pan. Place the bread into the egg mixture. Turn over to coat on both sides. Set aside to allow the liquid to absorb.

Heat a griddle, skillet, or electric frying pan. Melt 1 tablespoon butter until foaming. Shake gently to coat the cooking surface. Add the bread and dust with cinnamon. When the undersides are lightly browned, use a metal spatula to turn. Add more butter, if needed.

Remove and set aside to keep warm. Add more butter to the griddle for the remaining slices.

Serve immediately and top each serving with warm Strawberry Sauce.

YIELD: 4 SERVINGS

HEALTHFUL HINT: Don't shortchange yourself by eating white bread. It has a fraction of the vitamins and minerals contained in whole grain breads, and very little fiber. When whole grains are refined, 22 essential nutrients are removed, and 4 to 6 nutrients are replaced. White bread is then called "enriched".

Aunt Priscilla's Apricot-Barley Cereal with Grilled Apples

This heartland hot cereal is a great way to start off the day—especially on cold winter mornings. It will satisfy any savage sweet tooth!

In a 2-quart saucepan, combine the barley, salt, nutmeg, and cardamom. Dry roast on medium heat, until fragrant, about 2 minutes. Stir frequently to avoid burning.

Carefully add the apple juice, 1 cup water, apricots, cinnamon stick, and 2 teaspoons butter. Bring to a boil, covered, over medium high heat. Reduce heat, and simmer until the barley is tender and all the liquid has been absorbed, from 50 to 60 minutes.

Using the remaining ½ teaspoon butter, grease a 9- x 13-inch baking pan. Slice the apples crosswise into ¼-inch thin rounds, and place on the tray.

Position the oven rack 4 inches from the broiler heat source. Preheat the broiler.

In a small bowl, mix the maple syrup and 1 tablespoon water. Drizzle 1 tablespoon maple mixture on the apples and sprinkle with ⅛ teaspoon cinnamon. Broil until cooked, about 3 minutes.

Using a fork or metal spatula, turn the slices over and sprinkle with remaining maple mixture and cinnamon. Broil for 2 more minutes. The apples will be golden brown.

Spoon barley cereal into bowls and top with apple slices. Serve hot.

YIELD: 4 SERVINGS

HEALTHFUL HINT: Barley contains a substance that in studies has been shown to lower cholesterol.

1 cup barley

½ teaspoon sea salt

⅛ teaspoon nutmeg

⅛ teaspoon cardamom powder

2 cups unsweetened apple juice

1 cup plus 1 tablespoon purified water

¼ cup dried apricots, unsulphured preferred

1 cinnamon stick

2 ½ teaspoons unsalted butter

2 baking apples, core removed

1 tablespoon real maple syrup

¼ teaspoon cinnamon

Blueberry Pancakes with Creamy Fruit Topping

Who doesn't like blueberry pancakes? With a simple substitution of whole wheat flour, and with its bran and germ, you can increase your vitamin and fiber intake. It is much more nutritious than refined white flour.

1 ½ cups whole wheat pastry flour (see Note)

1 teaspoon baking powder

Pinch sea salt

1 ½ cups plain yogurt or buttermilk with active cultures

1 egg, organic preferred

½ teaspoon real vanilla extract (optional)

¼ to ½ cup blueberries

Unsalted butter

1 recipe Creamy Fruit Topping (see page 170)

½ cup real maple syrup

NOTE: Whole wheat pastry flour is lighter than regular whole wheat flour. We recommend it for pancakes and baked goods.

On low heat, begin warming a pancake griddle, skillet, or electric frying pan.

In a large bowl, combine the flour, baking powder, and salt.

Using a blender or whisk, mix the yogurt or buttermilk, egg, and vanilla. Add to the flour mixture, stirring just until the dry ingredients are moistened. Gently fold in the blueberries.

Increase the griddle heat to medium-high. Grease cooking surface with melted butter. For each pancake, ladle ¼ cup batter onto griddle. Cook until bubbles break through the top and undersides are lightly browned. Use a metal spatula to flip the pancakes, and cook until lightly browned.

Stack the cooked pancakes on a heat-proof dish, and keep warm. Continue making pancakes until all the batter has been used.

Serve a stack of 2 or 3 pancakes topped with 2 tablespoons Creamy Fruit Topping. Drizzle with maple syrup.

YIELD: 8 TO 12 PANCAKES

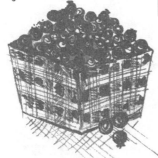

HEALTHFUL HINT: Whole wheat pastry flour is the equivalent of white refined cake or cuit flour plus the bran and germ. It has a nuttier flavor, and all of its nutrients are still in Substitute whole wheat pastry flour in your favorite recipes to give them added nutrition.

Spicy Turkey Patties on English Muffins

Reminiscent of pork sausage patties, but with less fat and calories—these can be enjoyed with little or no guilt!

In a blender or food processor, pulse chop the onion, garlic, and parsley.

Place them in a medium bowl and combine with the turkey, salt, spices, bread crumbs, and egg. Mix well.

Refrigerate for 10 to 15 minutes or overnight to allow flavors to blend.

In a large skillet, heat the oil or butter over a medium flame. Shape the turkey mixture into 8 patties and place in the skillet. Cook the patties until golden brown on both sides, about 2 minutes per side. If you prefer them crisper, cover the pan and continue cooking the patties another 6 minutes, turning occasionally.

Drain on brown paper or paper toweling.

Toast the English muffins. Place a patty on each half and serve the sandwiches open-faced. Serve while hot.

YIELD: 4 SERVINGS

HEALTHFUL HINT: Lifting a heavy skillet by the handle can add a great deal of strain to your hands and arms. Instead, look into purchasing skillet "clip-on" handles that allow you disperse the weight evenly between your two hands—without getting burned.

1 onion, peeled and quartered

2 cloves garlic, peeled

4 sprigs fresh parsley, thick stems removed and washed

½ pound lean ground turkey

½ teaspoon herbal sea salt

½ teaspoon thyme

½ teaspoon red pepper flakes

¼ teaspoon sage

¼ teaspoon ginger powder

¼ teaspoon cardamom powder

¼ teaspoon ground black pepper

1 tablespoon whole grain bread crumbs

1 egg, organic preferred, lightly beaten

2 tablespoons extra virgin olive oil or ghee

4 whole grain English muffins

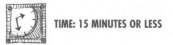

Frittata and Omelette Primer with Toppings and Fillings

Omelettes and frittatas are fast and easy to make (see note). They offer a hearty protein base for savory, spicy, or rich fillings and toppings. Serve them along with toasted whole grain breads and a side of potatoes. For a real country breakfast, add a Spicy Turkey Patty (page 35), along with a cup of hot herbal tea.

8 eggs, organic preferred

½ teaspoon herbal sea salt

2 to 3 tablespoons unsalted butter

Any filling or topping desired (see Toppings and Fillings on the next page).

NOTE: The difference between the French omelette and the Italian frittata is that omelettes are folded over their fillings and frittatas are served open–faced.

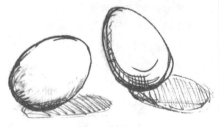

TO MAKE A FRITTATA:

Preheat the broiler. In a bowl or blender, lightly beat the eggs and salt.

Melt the butter in a 12-inch omelette pan over medium heat. Tilt the skillet in all directions to cover the entire bottom with butter and about ⅓ of the way up the sides.

Raise the heat to medium-high and pour in the eggs. Cook without stirring until the eggs begin to bubble around the edges, about 10 seconds. Stir the center, being careful not to pierce the bottom and to keep it in one piece. Continue cooking about 3 minutes.

Place the skillet under the broiler for 2-3 minutes, or until frittata is puffed and golden.

Carefully slide the frittata out of the skillet and onto a plate. Cover the top with any warm toppings and serve hot.

TO MAKE AN OMELETTE:

In a bowl or blender, lightly beat 2 eggs and salt.

Melt 1 tablespoon butter in a 6- or 8-inch omelette pan (a skillet with slopping sides), over medium heat. Tilt the skillet in all directions to cover the entire bottom with butter and about ⅓ of the way up the sides.

Raise the heat and pour in the eggs. Cook without stirring until the eggs begin to bubble around the edges, about 10 seconds. Stir the center, being careful not to pierce the bottom and to keep it in one piece. It should take about 1 minute for the bottom to set.

Place desired filling on half of the omelette. Carefully slide the omelet halfway onto the plate, then flip the other half over the bottom portion to form a half circle.

Place the plate in a warm oven and repeat for the 3 other omelettes (or use 4 omelette pans).

YIELD: 4 SERVINGS

Toppings and Fillings

Frittatas can be topped and omelettes filled with an amazing variety of ingredients. Be creative—how can you go wrong? Here are a few suggestions.

- **Caramelized onions and golden potatoes, with parsley and garlic.**
- **Avocado, fresh tomato, and chives.**
- **Sautéed red and green peppers, and garlic.**
- **Chèvre with herbs, walnuts, and scallions.**
- **Button, porcini, and oyster mushrooms sautéed with shallots.**
- **Sautéed leeks with salmon and fresh basil.**
- **Red onion, black olives, and anchovies.**

And Recipes from this Book (a great way to use leftovers):

- **Hearty Hummus** *(page 78)*
- **Cilantro Salsa** *(page 79)*
- **Kale with Capers and Pine Nuts** *(page 98)*
- **Italian Baked Asparagus** *(page 103)*
- **Curried Cauliflower with Cashews** *(page 100)*
- **Nutty Mushroom Pâté** *(page 47)*
- **Sweet Potato Aioli** *(page 52)*
- **Texas-Inspired Chili** *(page 115)*
- **The Tangiest Teriyaki Chicken** *(page 127)*

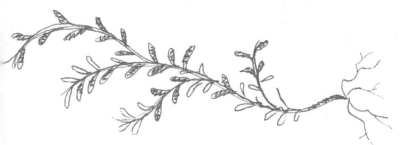

Russian Sunflower-Rye Muffins

Not just for the birds, sunflower seeds provide lots of valuable nutrients. These muffins freeze well.

1 cup rye flour (see Note)

½ cup whole wheat pastry flour

¼ cup currants, unsulphured preferred

1 tablespoon baking powder

½ teaspoon caraway seeds (optional)

½ teaspoon cinnamon

½ teaspoon sea salt

1 cup plain yogurt with active cultures or buttermilk

½ cup purified water or unsweetened apple juice

¼ cup unsalted butter, room temperature

3 tablespoons unsulphured blackstrap molasses

1 egg, organic preferred

2 to 4 tablespoons real maple syrup, or to taste

½ cup plus 2 tablespoons raw sunflower seeds, shelled and unsalted

NOTE: If rye flour is unavailable, substitute additional whole wheat pastry flour in equal proportions.

PREHEAT THE OVEN TO 350 DEGREES.

Prepare muffin tins with paper inserts. In a large bowl combine the rye and pastry flours, currants, baking powder, caraway, cinnamon, and salt.

Using a blender or food processor, mix the yogurt, water, butter, molasses, egg, and maple syrup. Add ½ cup sunflower seeds and pulse blend 2 to 3 seconds.

Make a well in the center of the dry ingredients, and add yogurt mixture. Stir just until the dry ingredients are moistened. Do not over mix.

Spoon the batter into the prepared muffin tins, filling cups three-quarters full. Sprinkle tops with the remaining seeds.

Bake the muffins until the tops are golden and centers test done, about 20 minutes.

Transfer the muffins to a cooling rack.

YIELD: 9 TO 12 MUFFINS

HEALTHFUL HINT: Blackstrap molasses, a by-product of sugar refining, is high in lots of minerals, especially calcium and iron. Purchase the unsulphured kind to avoid the added sulphur dioxide.

TIME: 35 MINUTES

Coconut-Orange Muffins with Walnuts

Tropical tasting yet fully grounded in good nutrition, these make a terrific breakfast or snack. Keep some handy in the freezer.

PREHEAT THE OVEN TO 350 DEGREES.

Prepare muffin tins with paper inserts. In a large bowl, combine the pastry flour, coconut, baking powder, cinnamon, ginger, and salt.

In blender or food processor, whip the butter until soft. Add the yogurt, maple syrup, molasses, and egg, mixing well. Mix in the orange zest and juice.

Pour the butter mixture into the flour and using a fork, stir until moistened.

Spoon the batter into the muffin cups ³/₄ full. Cover the tops with walnuts. Bake until the tops are golden, about 15 to 20 minutes.

Transfer the muffins to a cooling rack.

YIELD: 9 TO 12 MUFFINS

HEALTHFUL HINT: Skipping breakfast may save you calories at first, but can lead to weight gain when hunger comes later on and rampant eating occurs. Fuel yourself for the action of the day with a meal that contains starch-protein and fats for a long energy haul.

1 ½ cups whole wheat pastry flour

½ cup unsweetened coconut

1 tablespoon baking powder

1 teaspoon cinnamon

½ teaspoon ground ginger

½ teaspoon sea salt

½ cup unsalted butter, room temperature

1 cup buttermilk or plain yogurt with active cultures

½ cup real maple syrup or honey

¼ cup blackstrap molasses, unsulphured preferred

1 egg, organic preferred

1 orange, zest and juice, organic preferred, or

1 teaspoon orange extract

1 cup raw walnuts

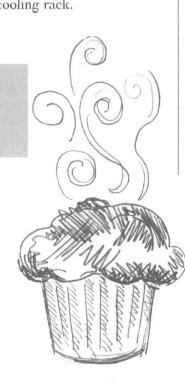

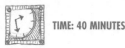

Southwestern Corn Bread

Most people think that cornbread is full of fat. Not this version. A great companion for eggs at breakfast, serve it with our Texas-Inspired Chili (page 115) or Yummy Red Lentil Soup (page 84) for lunch or dinner.

1 or 2 carrots, washed, trimmed, and quartered

¾ cup high-lysine cornmeal

¾ cup whole wheat pastry flour

½ cup plus 2 tablespoons raw sunflower seeds, shelled and unsalted

2 teaspoons baking powder

½ teaspoon sea salt

2 tablespoons unsalted butter, room temperature

2 eggs, organic preferred

¼ cup real maple syrup or honey

1 cup plain yogurt with active cultures or buttermilk

PREHEAT THE OVEN TO 425 DEGREES.

Grease an 8-inch square baking pan, round cast iron skillet, or an 8-cup muffin tin.

Using a blender or food processor, pulse chop the carrots. Remove carrots to a medium bowl and add the cornmeal, flour, ½ cup sunflower seeds, baking powder, and salt, and stir to distribute evenly.

Without cleaning blender or processor, add butter and puree. Add eggs and maple syrup or honey, and mix well.

Make a well in the carrot-cornmeal mixture and add butter blend. Pour the yogurt or buttermilk on top and stir until the dry ingredients are just moistened. Do not over mix.

Pour or spoon the batter into the prepared pan or muffin cups. Sprinkle tops with remaining sunflower seeds. Bake until a toothpick inserted in the center comes out clean and the top is golden, about 20 to 25 minutes.

YIELD: ONE 8- X 8-INCH BREAD OR 8 MUFFINS

HEALTHFUL HINT: Eating a variety of grains provides your body with different nutrients than the ususal wheat and rice. This cornbread is a way to fill your baked goods with nourishing ingredients, and is a terrific wholesome meal on-the-run.

Shrimp and Swiss Chard Scramble with Pineapple Garnish

Perfect for breakfast or brunch, this rich-tasting, low-fat egg dish is an ideal addition to your repertoire—and a clever way to put greens into your day.

Place the Swiss chard and water in a medium-sized sauté pan over medium heat. Cover and steam until wilted, about 5 minutes. Drain and rinse with cold water to cool.

Using a blender or food processor, pulse chop the onion.

Rinse the sauté pan (from cooking the Swiss chard). Place over medium heat, add butter and melt. Add the onions and sauté until soft, about 5 minutes.

Meanwhile, press or squeeze the water out of the chard. Place in blender or processor and pulse chop. Add chopped greens to the onions and stir, allowing the chard to dry a little. Add the shrimp, salt, and pepper. Cook until the shrimp turns pink and vegetables are hot, about 2 to 3 minutes.

Pour eggs into the skillet and mix together with the shrimp mixture. Cook over medium heat, until eggs are lightly set.

Spoon onto a large platter and garnish with pineapple or mango slices.

YIELD: 4 SERVINGS

½ bunch Swiss chard or spinach, washed, about 1 cup

½ cup purified water

1 to 2 onions, peeled and quartered (see Note)

2 tablespoons unsalted butter

½ pound small-size raw shrimp, peeled and deveined

Pinch sea salt

Pinch ground pepper

4 eggs, organic preferred, lightly beaten

Fresh pineapple or papaya slices, for garnish

NOTE: If you're without a machine to chop onions, you can use 1 to 2 tablespoons of dry onion flakes per onion. What you will be missing is the antioxidant and HDL-cholesterol boosts of the fresh onion.

HEALTHFUL HINT: Fresh pineapple contains bromelain, an enzyme with anti-inflammatory properties which can reduce pain caused by arthritis. Papaya also contains digestive enzymes, and is a rich source of vitamins C and A, and potassium. Because enzymes are destroyed by heat, it is important to eat these fruits raw rather than cooked.

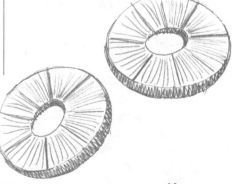

South of France Chicken and Olive Sandwiches

Sandwiches are great for a light lunch or a summer entrée. Serve with a bowl of hot soup such as Purely Simple Egg Drop Soup (page 85), for a more filling meal.

1 ½ tablespoons extra virgin olive oil

1 onion, peeled and sliced

1 teaspoon basil, dried, or 2 tablespoons fresh, chopped leaves

1 lemon, organic preferred, zest and juice

¼ teaspoon red pepper flakes

¼ teaspoon sea salt

3 tablespoons purified water

4 chicken cutlet breasts, organic preferred, skinless and sliced thin

10 Greek or Kalamata olives, pitted, or 3 tablespoons olive paste

8 slices crusty whole grain bread

Prepared mustard

4 Boston or romaine lettuce leaves

1 large ripe tomato, thinly sliced

Hot sauce (optional)

NOTE: Greek or Kalamata olives are softer and easier to pit by hand than many smaller varieties.

Heat a medium-sized skillet on a moderate flame. Add 1 tablespoon oil and onion, and cook until slightly softened, about 4 minutes.

Add the basil, lemon zest, pepper flakes, and salt. Stir to combine. Cover and cook another 5 minutes. Remove to a small bowl.

Add remaining ½ tablespoon oil and water to pan, and stir to incorporate the flavors from cooking the onions. Add the chicken cutlets and season with a pinch of salt and lemon juice. Cook until tender, about 5 to 6 minutes on each side.

Coarsely chop the olives. Place in a small bowl. Toast or grill the bread.

To assemble, place 4 slices of bread on a work surface. Smear each with mustard and place a lettuce leaf and a slice of tomato on top. Layer with a chicken cutlet, the cooked onions, and sprinkle with chopped olives (or spread the olive paste on the top slice of toast). Sprinkle each sandwich with a little hot sauce, if desired. Top with the second bread slice. Cut the sandwich in half on the diagonal.

YIELD: 4 SERVINGS

HEALTHFUL HINT: Whole grain breads provide vitamin E and selenium, two important antioxidants, that protect cells from free radicals, Selenium can also help to keep the immune system functioning properly.

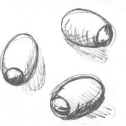

Avocado and Watercress Pita with Garlic-Onion Jam

Avocados are a great tasting food to include in your meals and are available year-round.

Place avocado slices on a plate and set aside. Dry the watercress on a cotton cloth or paper toweling.

Cut the pita breads in half. Place them in the toaster oven to soften and warm, about 30 seconds.

To assemble, spread some Garlic-Onion Jam on one side of each pita half. Stuff in 2 or 3 tender stems of watercress, 2 or 3 slices of avocado, and a slice of red onion.

Serve 2 pita halves per person with a lemon wedge and pickle on the side. Everyone can squeeze their own lemon onto the sandwiches.

YIELD: 4 SERVINGS

2 ripe avocados, peeled, pitted, and sliced

1 bunch watercress, washed, and thick stems removed

4 whole grain pita breads

1 recipe Garlic-Onion Jam (page 166)

1 red onion, peeled and thinly sliced

Lemon wedges

4 dill pickles

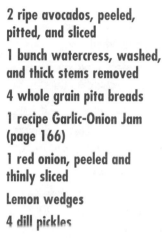

HEALTHFUL HINT: The primary source for the antioxidant vitamin E are vegetable oils. Avocados and whole grain breads are two foods that contain this important free radical antidote. Sunflower seeds, walnuts, almonds, prunes, and peaches are some other foods that contain vitamin E.

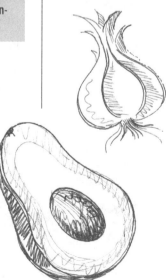

Open-faced Tuna Steak Sandwiches with Sun-dried Tomato Mayonnaise

Easy to cook and assemble, this wonderful sandwich offers you taste, texture, and style. Your friends will be amazed.

1 tablespoon extra virgin olive oil

2 boneless tuna steaks, cut 1- 1 ½ inches thick

Herbal sea salt

1 teaspoon balsamic vinegar

4 slices whole grain sourdough bread

1 recipe Sun-dried Tomato Mayonnaise (page 168)

4 beautiful green or red leaf lettuce leaves

1 bunch arugula, thick stems removed and washed

1 cup fresh radish sprouts (see Note)

NOTE: Radish sprouts are quite spicy and can add zip to any recipe that calls for sprouts.

Heat a large skillet over high heat. Add the oil, then add the tuna steaks. Sprinkle the tuna lightly with herbal salt. Cook for 2 minutes. Using a spatula, carefully turn the steaks over. Sprinkle again with herbal salt, and drizzle a little vinegar on each. Continue to cook another 3 minutes, for medium rare. Set on a plate to cool slightly.

Toast or grill the bread. Arrange the toast on individual plates and cover each with a thick layer of Sun-dried Tomato Mayonnaise, and then a lettuce leaf and several stems of arugula.

Cut the tuna into slices, and place on top of the greens. Top the sandwiches with a loose bunch of sprouts. Drizzle a little vinegar on the sprouts, and serve with a knife and fork.

YIELD: 4 SERVINGS

HEALTHFUL HINT: Tuna is a rich source of eicosapentaenoic acid (EPA), the best known of the omega-3 fatty acids, which can help reduce arthritic inflammation.

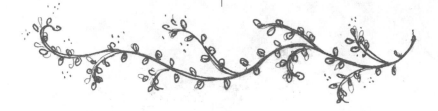

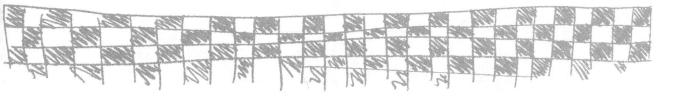

Appetizers, Snacks, and Small Meals

Avocado and Red Onion Guacamole

Nutty Mushroom Pâté

Mediterranean Cucumber Tzatziki

Curry Nut Mix

Bruschetta Italiana

Salmon Spread

Sweet Potato Aioli

Yogurt and Scallion Cheese

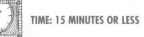

Avocado and Red Onion Guacamole

When ripened, Haas avocados are black and Florida avocados are green, and both are slightly soft to a gentle squeeze. This dip makes a great addition to any meal, and thinned with a little water becomes a wonderful salad dressing. Try stuffing this dip into a whole wheat pita for a hearty snack or small meal.

½ red onion, peeled and cut in half

1 clove garlic, peeled

2 ripe avocados

2 to 3 tablespoons lemon juice

½ teaspoon sea salt

Baked corn chips or whole wheat pita toast points (page 80)

In a blender or food processor, pulse mince the onion and garlic.

Cut the avocados in half, remove the pits, and set them aside. Using a spoon, scoop the avocado flesh out. Put into the processor with the onion and garlic. Add the lemon and salt. Blend just enough to mix or puree completely.

Place the guacamole in a serving bowl, and place the pits in it. (This keeps the avocado from turning brown.) Place the corn chips or pita in a basket, and munch away.

YIELD: 4 SERVINGS

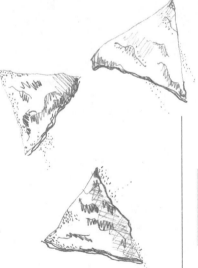

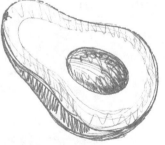

HEALTHFUL HINT: Although avocados contain a lot of fat, it is the beneficial mono-unsaturated kind that's also in olive oil. It also has vitamin E, folic acid, and potassium—all of which are inflammation busters.

Nutty Mushroom Pâté

Many meat pâtés are just brimming with fat and calories. This tasty, low-fat alternative is rich and flavorful, much like its cholesterol-laden cousins, but this pâté is full of joint-smart foods and spices. Enjoy!

Grind ½ cup walnuts or almonds in a blender or food processor. Place the ground nuts in a mixing bowl and set aside.

Using the same machine (don't worry if there are a few nut particles left in it), pulse chop the onion and garlic.

Heat the oil or butter in a large skillet, over a medium flame. Add the onion and garlic, and cook uncovered, until tender, about 5 minutes. Stir occasionally.

Add the mushrooms, thyme, salt, and pepper. Cook over medium heat, covered, until mushrooms are tender and aromatic, about 15 minutes. Stir often. Uncover and continue cooking until the mushroom water evaporates, another 2 to 3 minutes.

Rinse blender or processor bowl. Add the mushroom sauté, and puree. Pour into the bowl with the ground nuts and stir mixture together. Taste and adjust salt and pepper. (A pâté's flavor reduces once chilled, thus it requires stronger seasoning while warm to be just right when cool.)

Spoon pâté into an oiled loaf pan. Cover with plastic wrap, and refrigerate for several hours.

Unmold onto a serving platter. Garnish with reserved nuts and parsley or sage.

YIELD: 1 LOAF

½ cup raw walnuts or almonds, plus 4 beautiful walnut halves or almonds (see Note)

1 onion, peeled and quartered

2 cloves garlic, peeled

2 tablespoons extra virgin olive oil or unsalted butter

1 pound button mushrooms, cleaned

½ teaspoon dried thyme

¼ to ½ teaspoon sea salt or herbal salt

Ground white pepper

Fresh parsley or sage sprigs for garnish

NOTE: For a richer taste, the walnuts or almonds can be toasted. Place the nuts in a pan and pop them into the toaster oven for 5 to 7 minutes. Be careful the nuts don't burn.

HEALTHFUL HINT: Onions are a source of joint-protective antioxidants. When choosing onions, pick yellow and red over white, because these have higher levels of antioxidants.

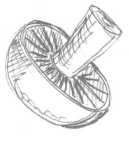
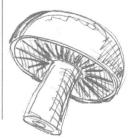

Mediterranean Cucumber Tzatziki

Serve this salad with chunks of whole grain bread or sesame pita triangles. It is also delicious as a topping on steamed vegetables, as a sandwich spread instead of mayonnaise, topping for a baked potato, or swirled into your favorite soup—the possibilities are endless!

2 Kirby or wax cucumbers, peeled

½ teaspoon sea salt

4 to 6 leaves fresh mint (see Note)

2 cloves garlic, peeled

2 cups plain yogurt with active cultures

1 tablespoon extra virgin olive oil

European whole grain bread

NOTE: Forgot the fresh mint? Use a mint tea bag—just open one up and stir it in.

Place a colander over a bowl or in the sink. Cut the cucumbers lengthwise and then in quarters. Sprinkle the spears with salt and toss to coat. Let the cucumbers stand for 15 minutes to drain.

Run water briefly over the cumbers to remove salt. Shake colander to remove excess water.

In a blender or food processor, pulse chop the mint and garlic. Add the yogurt and oil, and blend briefly until smooth and creamy. Pour into a large bowl.

Pulse chop the cucumbers and add to the yogurt. Mix the ingredients well.

Serve at room temperature or chill, if preferred. Taste and adjust seasoning, if needed.

Serve with hunks or slices of European bread.

YIELD: 4 SERVINGS

HEALTHFUL HINT: If you tend to get digestive gas when eating cucumbers, use this method of salting them, and they will become more digestible.

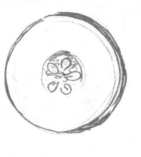

Curry Nut Mix

Nuts are an ideal way to include the essential fatty acids (EFAs) in our daily diets. EFAs are important since they are one of the components of our tissues, organs, and glands. These healthful EFAs also help to reduce inflammation.

In a large sauté pan on medium heat, melt the butter or oil. Add the curry powder and cook, just until it begins to bubble, about 30 seconds.

Add the nuts and seeds, and cook until lightly browned, stirring constantly, about 3 to 5 minutes.

Immediately transfer to a wide bowl or plate. Stir in the currants, if desired. Cool before eating or storing.

YIELD: 2 ½ CUPS

2 tablespoons unsalted butter or extra virgin olive oil

2 teaspoons curry powder

2 cups raw mixed nuts and seeds, including almonds, cashews, walnuts, sunflower seeds, and pumpkin seeds

½ cup currants, unsulphured preferred (optional)

HEALTHFUL HINT: Curry is an ideal flavor choice in an arthritis-sensitive diet because it can be made from a mixture of spices — cinnamon, clove, turmeric, ginger — known to reduce the swelling in joints. Choose a curry powder that suits your tastes, as they can be purchased mild and sweet tasting to hot and spicy.

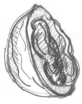

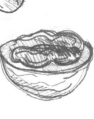

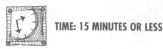 **TIME: 15 MINUTES OR LESS**

Bruschetta Italiana

A fancy name for slices of toasted bread with a topping that can be served as is, broiled, or baked. Serve alone or alongside a bowl of warm and friendly soup. A real treat without much effort!

4 slices whole grain bread either from a baguette, a pre-sliced loaf, or miniature pita breads

Toast the bread and then top with your choice of the following:

- Rub peeled raw garlic on toasted bread and drizzle with extra virgin olive oil, then sprinkle with oregano and a tiny bit of herbal salt.
- A smear of cashew nut butter topped with avocado slices, and a few drops of lemon.
- Rub peeled raw garlic on toast and top with a slice or two of tomato.
- Spread with Nutty Mushroom Pâté (page 47) and top with crumbled goat or feta cheese.
- Butter toast and sprinkle with grated parmesan cheese and minced parsley.
- Smear with tahini and apple butter.

Eat as is, or broil or bake for several minutes until the topping begins to bubble.

YIELD: 4 SERVINGS

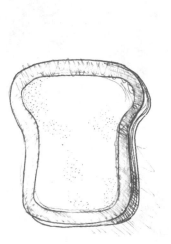

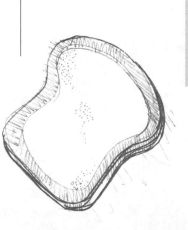

HEALTHFUL HINT: This savory Italian toast is usually made with white bread, which is missing the full range of nutrients that are in whole grain breads. Look for specialty bakeries that bake wonderfully flavorful loaves and baguettes made with whole grains, and give yourself a full complement of vitamins and minerals when you enjoy this appetizer. Buy an extra loaf, and keep it in the freezer.

Salmon Spread

Here's a way to add a light protein and essential fatty acids to a small meal, with a smear of this great tasting fish spread.

Place the salmon and water in a small frying pan. Bring to a boil, covered, lower flame and cook until tender when pierced with a fork, about 5 to 7 minutes. Drain in a colander. Place the drained fish on a plate, and using a fork, flake it into large pieces. Allow to cool, about 5 minutes.

In a blender or food processor, combine the salmon, yogurt, dill, horseradish, salt, and pepper until smooth. Serve with crackers or spread on your favorite whole grain bread.

YIELD: 2 CUPS

¼ pound fresh salmon, skinned

Purified water

1 cup plain yogurt with active cultures

2 sprigs fresh dill

1 teaspoon prepared or ½ teaspoon freshly grated horseradish

¼ teaspoon sea salt

½ teaspoon ground white pepper

HEALTHFUL HINT: The most effective type of omega-3 fatty acids are the EPAs, which are found in salmon and are the best natural inflammation fighters. We recommend eating fish 2 to 5 times per week. What a delightful way to incorporate your fish servings!

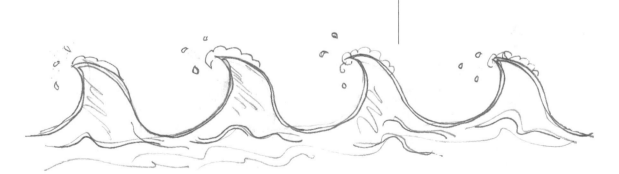

Sweet Potato Aioli

A great use for already baked sweet potatoes or yams. When baking potatoes, cook a couple of extra ones and make this dish the next day.

2 large sweet potatoes or yams, baked (see Note)

6 to 8 cloves garlic, peeled

¼ cup extra virgin olive oil

¼ cup flaxseed oil

1 tablespoon fresh lemon juice

2 tablespoons purified water

Hot pepper sauce, to taste (optional)

1 teaspoon sea salt

Ground black pepper

NOTE: To bake the potatoes; preheat the oven to 400 degrees. Place the sweet potatoes or yams on a baking tray and bake until soft when pierced with a fork, about 50 minutes. Remove from the oven and set aside until cool enough to handle.

Peel the potatoes and cut into chunks. Mince the garlic in a blender or food processor. Add the sweet potatoes and process until very smooth. A little at a time, add the olive and flax oils, lemon juice, and water. Using a rubber spatula, scrap down the sides of the machine bowl. Add the hot pepper sauce, salt, and pepper and process until everything is well blended.

Serve at room temperature.

YIELD: 2 CUPS

HEALTHFUL HINT: Researchers have found that the carotenoids (beta carotene, the plant form of vitamin A, is one of many) are very effective in fighting free radicals, the unstable molecules that roam around the body attacking and destroying healthy tissue and joints. Yellow-orange vegetables such as these sweet potatoes, and fruits, as well as dark leafy greens are a good source of carotenoids.

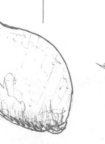

Yogurt and Scallion Cheese

Here's an inventive way to include protein, calcium, and beneficial active cultures that promote better digestion and nutrient assimilation. And it's unbelievably great tasting! Spread some on toast for a small meal or snack.

Drain the yogurt for 2 hours or overnight, refrigerated. (see Note)

In a blender or food processor, pulse mince the scallions, garlic, and parsley. Pour into a medium bowl. Add the drained yogurt, salt, and pepper, and mix well.

YIELD: 2 CUPS

4 scallions, trimmed and cut in quarters

1 clove garlic, peeled

4 sprigs fresh parsley, thick stems removed

2 cups plain yogurt with active cultures

¼ teaspoon herbal sea salt

⅛ teaspoon ground pepper

HEALTHFUL HINT: The yogurt we recommend has active cultures that are beneficial to digestion and assimilation. We can't say enough about eating this wonderful-for-you food.

NOTE: Place a colander in a bowl and line it with paper coffee filters or several layers of cheesecloth. Pour the yogurt into the lined colander and put it in the refrigerator to drain for 2 hours or overnight.

"Food is our common ground, a universal experience."

—James Beard

Accompaniments and Side Dishes

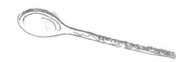

Arroz Olé

Midwestern Cornmeal Wedges

Sweet and Savory Curried Rice Pulao

Russian Mushroom Kasha

Savory Saffron Couscous

Mashed Sweet Potatoes

Quinoa with Roasted Garlic and Pignoli Nuts

Babe's Real Greek Pilaf

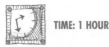
Arroz Olé

This spicy Latin-inspired variation on a traditional rice pilaf is an exciting addition to any meal. Try serving it with one of our many seafood dishes or as a tasty complement to a chicken entree.

2 ½ cups chicken or vegetable stock, homemade preferred, or purified water

½ teaspoon saffron threads

1 onion, peeled and quartered

3 cloves garlic, peeled

2 tablespoons extra virgin olive oil or unsalted butter

1 green pepper, seeded

1 cup brown rice, washed (see Whole Grain Facts, page 199)

½ teaspoon sea salt

¼ teaspoon red pepper flakes (optional)

¼ teaspoon ground black pepper

In a medium-sized saucepan bring the stock to a boil, covered. Add saffron and simmer for several minutes. Using a food processor fitted with a slicing blade, slice the onion and garlic.

In a large skillet or sauce pan, heat 1 tablespoon oil or butter over medium heat. Add the onions and garlic, and sauté uncovered, until onions have softened, about 5 minutes.

Meanwhile, using the processor, slice the peppers.

Add the remaining 1 tablespoon oil or butter and the rice. Sauté until rice begins to brown and smell roasted. Stir frequently, being careful not to burn the rice.

Carefully add the stock. Add the salt, pepper flakes, and pepper, and stir once. Bring to a boil, covered, reduce heat to low and simmer until all the liquid is absorbed and the rice is tender, about 50 minutes.

YIELD: 4 SERVINGS

HEALTHFUL HINT: Whole grains, such as the brown rice in this recipe, with its bran and germ intact, contain all the major nutrient groups — carbohydrates, protein, fat, vitamins, minerals, and fiber. White rice has been stripped of most of these vital nutrients — so why bother using it?

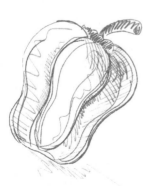

Midwestern Cornmeal Wedges

Otherwise known as cornmeal mush, grits, or polenta, this wonderful dish can be prepared days in advance. Served hot and soft, it's a great breakfast cereal. Cooled, cornmeal can be molded and cut into wedges or slices.

Put the water in a medium-sized saucepan, and whisk in the cornmeal and salt. Bring to a boil, stirring frequently to prevent cornmeal from settling on the bottom of the pot. At first use the whisk, and as it thickens change to a wooden spoon.

Reduce heat, cover and simmer for 35 minutes. Stir occasionally. The cornmeal will be thick. If needed, add a small amount of water.

Turn off the flame. Add the butter and pepper. Cover for a minute to allow the butter to melt, then stir it in.

Under cold water, rinse the inside of a 9- or 10-inch mold, a round pie plate, or a loaf pan, leaving it wet. Pour the cornmeal in and set aside to cool, about 30 to 40 minutes. It will solidify as it cools.

When solidified, turn the mold onto a platter. Cut into wedges.

YIELD: 4 SERVINGS

3 cups purified water

1 cup high-lysine cornmeal, not instant or quick-cooking

1 teaspoon sea salt

2 tablespoons unsalted butter

½ teaspoon ground white pepper

NOTE: An alternative to cooking cornmeal from scratch is to buy it ready-made. In some stores you can now find sausage-shaped tubes of already prepared cornmeal or polenta. This can be cut into round slices and sautéed in butter for a tasty side-dish.

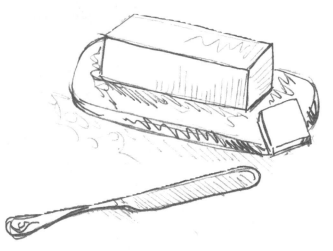

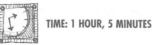

Sweet and Savory Curried Rice Pulao

You don't have to go out to an Indian restaurant to enjoy this flavorful rice dish from the East. Serve this as an entree course with our Eternal Life Seven Vegetable Stew (page 111), or as a delightful side dish with lamb or veal.

1 carrot, washed, trimmed, and quartered

2 tablespoons unsalted butter

2 tablespoons currants or raisins, unsulphured preferred

2 ½ cups chicken stock, homemade preferred, or purified water

1 cup long-grain brown rice, washed (see page 199)

½ teaspoon cinnamon

½ teaspoon cardamom powder

½ teaspoon ginger powder

½ teaspoon sea salt

¼ teaspoon nutmeg

¼ teaspoon mace

¼ teaspoon ground white pepper

PREHEAT THE OVEN TO 300 DEGREES. (CHECK SHELF HEIGHT TO MAKE SURE POT WILL FIT.)

In a small processor, coarsely chop the carrot. In a 2- to 3-quart Dutch oven, melt the butter over medium heat. Add the carrot and raisins. Sauté, until the carrot turns brownish around the edges, from 10 to 12 minutes. Stir frequently.

To the carrots, add the stock, rice, salt, and spices. Bring to a boil on high heat, covered.

Carefully place the pot in the oven and bake for 40 minutes.

Turn off oven heat and let pulao remain in oven for an additional 10 minutes.

Fluff the rice with a fork. Spoon onto a platter, and serve hot.

YIELD: 4 SERVINGS

HEALTHFUL HINT: Indian spices are known to ease swelling and inflammation and offer relief for arthritis.

"It's what you learn after you know it all that counts."

—John Wooden

Russian Mushroom Kasha

This easy-to-make, tasty dish will undoubtedly become one of your favorites. Try it along-side scrambled eggs for a hearty breakfast, or with a green salad and bean soup, for a satisfying dinner.

In a medium bowl mix the kasha, egg, and salt until the kasha is thoroughly coated.

Heat a 2-quart saucepan and add 2 teaspoons butter. Add the kasha mixture and cook briefly over high heat for about 2 minutes, stirring constantly. (This keeps the kasha from sticking together when cooking in the water.)

Carefully add the boiling water. Cover the pot and cook kasha over low heat until the liquid is absorbed, about 15 minutes.

Meanwhile, in a blender or food processor, pulse chop the onion. Heat a sauté pan on a medium flame with the remaining 2 teaspoons butter, and the onion. Pulse chop the mushrooms, and add to the pan along with the herbal salt and pepper. Sauté until softened, about 5 minutes.

Fluff the kasha with a fork and transfer to a serving bowl. Stir in the mushroom sauté and serve.

YIELD: 4 SERVINGS

HEALTHFUL HINT: Kasha is the only grain to contain bioflavonoids, which supports your body in building and maintaining collagen.

1 cup whole kasha (see page 203)

1 egg, organic preferred

½ teaspoon sea salt

4 teaspoons unsalted butter

2 cups purified water, boiling

1 onion, peeled and quartered

1 cup mushrooms

½ teaspoon herbal sea salt

¼ teaspoon pepper

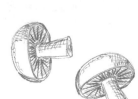

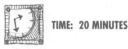

Savory Saffron Couscous

This dish is so great that it can be made over and over—even when Moroccan Tagine (page 113) is not on the menu.

3 cups purified water

1 teaspoon herbal sea salt

Several strands saffron

2 cloves garlic, peeled

1 onion, peeled and quartered

½ teaspoon cinnamon

¼ teaspoon coriander

8 to 10 oil-cured black olives, pitted

8 to 10 almonds

4 to 6 prunes, unsulphured preferred

4 to 6 pitted dates

1 ½ cups whole grain couscous

In a large saucepan, combine the water, salt, and saffron. Bring to a boil, covered. Reduce heat; simmer to allow saffron to dissolve, about 2 minutes.

In a blender or food processor, pulse chop the garlic and onion. Add to the saucepan and increase the flame to high.

Add the cinnamon, coriander, olives, almonds, prunes, and dates, and return the pot to a boil. Add the couscous and stir once. Cover the pot, lower flame, and simmer for 10 minutes.

Fluff with a fork. Transfer to a serving platter.

YIELD: 4 SERVINGS

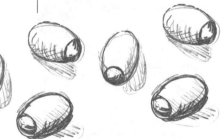

HEALTHFUL HINT: Couscous is a variety of pasta. The commercial variety is made with refined semolina flour. It is now easy to find whole grain couscous in natural food stores. It has a rich and nutty flavor, and cooks the same as its refined cousin.

Mashed Sweet Potatoes

What's so special about white potatoes and gravy? Try some of these updated spuds and you may never go back to their white cousins again!

PREHEAT THE OVEN TO 400 DEGREES.

Place the sweet potatoes or yams on a baking sheet and put into the oven. Bake until soft when pierced with a fork, about 45 to 55 minutes, depending on their size.

Remove potatoes from the oven and allow them to cool enough to handle, about 10 to 15 minutes.

Peel the skins off the potatoes and cut them into large chunks. Place the potatoes in a food processor and puree until smooth.

In a medium saucepan, heat the juice, butter, and salt. Add the potato puree and stir well. Heat thoroughly and serve.

YIELD: 4 SERVINGS

HEALTHFUL HINT: To give your body plenty of antioxidants everyday, eat at least one food from the carotenoids / vitamin A list. Yellow-orange fruits and vegetables such as apricots, sweet potatoes, pumpkin, carrots, cantaloupe, mangoes, peaches, yams, and winter squash are on the list as well as dark leafy greens such as broccoli, spinach, collard greens, parsley, and other leafy greens. These foods counteract free-radical damage to your joints and tissues.

4 sweet potatoes or yams, washed

¼ cup unsweetened apple juice or purified water

2 tablespoons unsalted butter or flaxseed oil

¼ to ½ teaspoon herbal sea salt

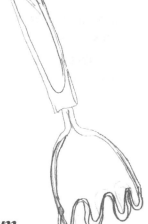

"Dice 'em, hash 'em, boil 'em, mash 'em! Idaho, Idaho, Idaho."

—Former Idaho football cheer

Quinoa with Roasted Garlic and Pignoli Nuts

This delicate and pearly grain, pronounced (KEEN-wah) has made an appearance in the American food scene. It originated in the Andes of South America and was an important part of the ancient Inca's diet. Use this dish alongside vegetable stew or meat loaf for a very satisfying meal.

1 head garlic

1 cup quinoa, washed (see page 199)

2 cups purified water

1 bay leaf

½ teaspoon basil

½ teaspoon sea salt

½ cup pignoli nuts

1 tablespoon unsalted butter or extra virgin olive oil

¼ teaspoon ground pepper or ⅛ teaspoon red pepper flakes

PREHEAT THE OVEN TO 400 DEGREES.

Place the bulb of garlic in a small baking pan, and put in the oven. Bake until the cloves are soft, about 25 to 30 minutes. (The garlic can be cooked the day before.)

Put the quinoa, water, bay leaf, basil, and salt in a 2-quart saucepan. Bring to a boil, covered. Reduce heat and simmer for 20 minutes.

Meanwhile, toast the pignoli nuts. Either place them in a small baking dish and toast in the oven while the garlic is roasting, or dry roast in a small frying pan on top of the stove. Either way, pignolis will toast quickly, in about 3 or 4 minutes. Stir frequently so they do not burn. After toasting, immediately remove the hot nuts to a small nonplastic bowl to cool.

Remove the garlic from the oven and allow to cool. Separate the cloves of garlic from their paper skins. A gentle squeeze will do it. Add them to the pignolis with the butter or oil and pepper, and stir.

Fluff the quinoa with a fork, and stir in the garlic-pignoli mixture. Scoop into a covered casserole and keep warm.

YIELD: 4 SERVINGS

Babe's Real Greek Pilaf

This is a recipe that's been handed down from a master "pilafi" maker. Here we use the long grain brown rice—worth the extra cooking time, since it is packed with nutrients and fiber that are good for arthritis. Try this recipe with some of the many whole grain rices on the market such as wild, wehani, basmati, black, rose, jasmine, or a mixture of long and short grain brown rice.

In a blender or food processor, pulse chop the onion. Heat a medium saucepan with the butter and oil, and add the onion, rice, and vermicelli. Sauté on a medium-high flame stirring frequently, until the rice and pasta start to toast and smell nutty, about 10 minutes.

Carefully add the stock, salt, and pepper. Bring to a boil, covered. Lower flame and simmer until all the liquid has absorbed, about 45 minutes.

Fluff the rice with a fork, place in a serving bowl and eat while hot.

YIELD: 4 SERVINGS

HEALTHFUL HINT: According to the Composition of Foods published by the USDA, when brown rice is compared with white—brown has 12% more protein, 33% more calcium, 5 times more vitamin B1, 67% more vitamin B2, 3 times more niacin, and 2 ½ times as much potassium and iron. It has 100% more vitamin E, as there is none left in white rice. This paints the picture—eat whole grains and add the precious nutrients your body needs.

1 onion, peeled and quartered

2 tablespoons unsalted butter

2 tablespoons extra virgin olive oil

1 cup long grain brown rice, washed (see page 199)

1 cup whole wheat vermicelli pasta

3 cups chicken stock, homemade preferred

½ teaspoon sea salt

¼ teaspoon ground black pepper

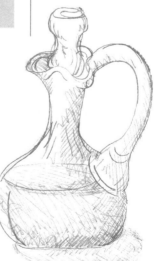

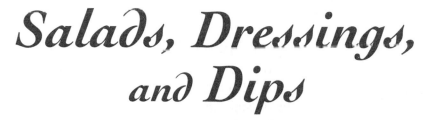

Salads, Dressings, and Dips

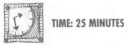
Mediterranean Taboule Grain Salad

This classic Mediterranean dish is full of herbs and spices that can soothe inflamed joints. Make it a day ahead of time, and the flavors have a chance to mingle.

1 cup purified water

½ cup bulghur wheat

½ teaspoon sea salt

2 cloves garlic, peeled

1 bunch parsley, thick stems removed

2 bunches scallions, quartered

6 fresh mint leaves (see Note)

4 fresh leaves or ½ teaspoon dry basil

½ cup extra virgin olive oil

½ cup lemon juice

¼ teaspoon ground pepper

1 Belgian endive, leaves separated

8 Greek olives, pitted

8 cherry tomatoes

NOTE: Forgot the fresh mint? Use a mint tea bag—just open one up and stir it into your salad.

In a 1-quart saucepan, bring the water to a boil. Add the bulghur and salt, cover and return to a boil. Turn off the flame, and set aside, allowing bulghur to absorb water and soften, about 15 minutes.

Using a blender or food processor, pulse chop the garlic, parsley, scallions, mint, and basil.

Fluff the bulghur with a fork and place in a medium bowl. Add the chopped herbs with the oil, lemon juice, and pepper. Taste and add additional salt, if desired.

Serve in a beautiful ceramic bowl garnished with endive spears, olives, and cherry tomatoes.

YIELD: 4 SERVINGS

HEALTHFUL HINT: Traditionally the herbs are all chopped by hand, which requires a lot of wrist action. Give yourself a break and chop your vegetables in the blender or food processor instead. For arthritis sufferers, it's a required piece of kitchen equipment!

Marinated Salmon Salad

This salad follows in the tradition of many gourmet offerings at trendy eateries. You can easily make fresh fish salad at home and enjoy all the fixings of a fancy lunch out — right in your own home.

RINSE THE SALMON IN COLD WATER AND DRY WITH PAPER TOWELS.

Bring the water to a boil in a large sauté pan over medium-high heat. Add the salmon and cover. Cook until the fish begins to flake and has no resistance to inserted fork, 5 to 7 minutes. Transfer the salmon to a large platter, and allow fish to cool.

In a blender or food processor, pulse chop the parsley, scallions, and garlic. Add these to the same sauté pan, with the lemon and lime juices, 1 tablespoon oil, and hot-pepper sauce. Cook for 1 to 2 minutes.

Using a fork, gently break up and flake the salmon, and place into a serving bowl. Add the garlic medley, pan juices, and the remaining 3 tablespoons oil. Toss gently, cover, and refrigerate until chilled, about 30 minutes.

Serve with crunchy cucumber and celery spears, whole wheat sesame crackers, or as an open-faced sandwich.

YIELD: 4 SERVINGS

HEALTHFUL HINT: One of the most powerful antioxidants is vitamin E, but it has even more potency when accompanied by selenium. This useful mineral is found in salmon and also tuna — good reasons to eat these classic foods which aid in the prevention and healing of arthritic joints.

1 pound salmon fillet, skin removed (see Note)

½ cup purified water

4 sprigs fresh parsley, thick stems removed

4 scallions, trimmed and quartered

3 cloves garlic, peeled

¼ cup lemon juice

¼ cup lime juice

4 tablespoons extra virgin olive oil

¼ teaspoon hot pepper sauce (optional)

Cucumber and celery spears, crackers or sliced bread

NOTE: Don't try to remove the skin from the raw salmon yourself. Ask your fish store to prepare the fillet this way. Or cook the salmon first and then remove the skin. It will separate very easily.

Scandinavian Beet and Apple Salad

Many people have found this salad an amazing substitute for the picnic staples—potato salad and cole slaw. The glow of the yellow apples glistens through the deep red of the beets, making it an unforgettable dish year round.

2 beets, washed and trimmed

Purified water

2 yellow apples, cored and cut in slices

½ cup plain yogurt with active cultures

2 tablespoons flax seed oil or extra virgin olive oil

1 teaspoon lemon juice

½ teaspoon herbal sea salt

¼ teaspoon dill

Place the beets in a pressure cooker or saucepan, and cover with water. Seal pressure cooker or cover saucepan. On high heat, bring to pressure or to a boil. Reduce flame and cook until beets are soft when pierced with a fork, 30 minutes in a pressure cooker or 55 minutes in a saucepan.

Bring pressure cooker down and open according to manufacturer's directions. Place beets in a large bowl of cold water. To peel the beets, take a beet into the palm of your hands, hold it under the water and slip the skin off. Place the beet on a plate, and peel the second one. Discard skins.

Using a fork, pierce a beet to keep it from rolling. With a paring knife, cut the beet in half, then quarters, then into slices. Repeat with the remaining beet. Place the sliced beets in a medium bowl.

Add apples to the beets. Toss with yogurt, oil, lemon juice, herbal salt, and dill.

Eat as is or chill for 30 minutes and serve.

YIELD: 4 SERVINGS

HEALTHFUL HINT: Don't waste effort cutting and slicing hard raw vegetables. Cook them first and then cut, as we did with the beets in this recipe. And in general, if it's not necessary to peel, don't. The skin provides fiber, and just under the skin are many vitamins and minerals that will be lost if peeled. (For this recipe, the beets taste better if they are peeled after cooking.)

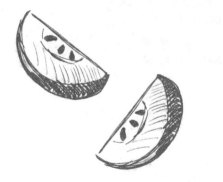
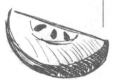
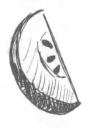

THE ARTHRITIS CURE COOKBOOK

Sassy Summer Fruit Salad

What's summer without fruit? This salad uses the best of fresh summer produce and gives it a sweet 'n spicy edge.

I n a blender or food processor, put almond butter, vinegar, honey, mustard, and salt. Puree until well blended. Add a little juice to thin, if desired.

Place the fruit in a glass serving bowl. Drizzle the sauce on top.

Serve at room temperature or chill briefly, if desired. Garnish with fresh mint sprigs.

YIELD: 4 SERVINGS

HEALTHFUL HINT: Berries are high in bioflavonoids and many minerals. These substances prevent cartilage from being destroyed when inflamed.

2 tablespoons raw almond butter (see Note)

1 teaspoon cider or wine vinegar

1 teaspoon real maple syrup or honey

⅛ teaspoon dry mustard

Pinch sea salt

Apple juice, as needed

3 to 4 cups blackberries, blueberries, and raspberries, or other favorite fruit

Fresh mint sprigs

NOTE: Almonds are rich with calcium and other minerals, have essential fatty acids that are good for your joints, and enough fat to give you that satisfied feeling. Almond butter is available in the natural food store. We recommend the raw, unsalted variety.

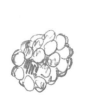

Quick and Easy Chinese Chicken Salad

This salad is the perfect—and healthy—way to make leftovers go the extra mile. Try it between slices of whole grain bread for a terrific sandwich.

½ cooked chicken (broiled, roasted, or boiled)

1 almond-sized knob fresh ginger

2 stalks celery, quartered

3 scallions, quartered

1 tablespoon imported soy sauce

Ground black pepper

2 tablespoons sesame or extra virgin olive oil

4 radishes

Remove the chicken meat from the bones, and cut into chunks (about 1 ½ cups). Place into a medium bowl.

In a blender or food processor, pulse chop the ginger. Add the celery and chop, then the scallions, chopping once more. Add to bowl with chicken.

Add the soy sauce, pepper, and oil. Toss together to mix. Serve at room temperature for best flavor. Serve with radishes on the side.

YIELD: 4 SERVINGS

HELPFUL HINT: Chicken contains a wide range of minerals—copper, manganese, phosphorus, potassium, zinc, calcium, and magnesium.

"A salad is not a meal. It is a style."

—Fran Lebowitz

Martini Salad

This citrus salad may seem unusual, but it's quite delicious and a perfect summer picnic treat. A great way to add bioflavonoids.

Using a paring knife, peel the oranges, leaving some traces of the pith (the white part). Cut oranges crosswise in ¼-inch thick slices and put in a medium bowl. Retain as much juice as possible. (Oranges may be sliced ahead of time, but do not blend with other ingredients until ready to serve, as the olives will stain them.)

In a small bowl combine the garlic, almond butter, salt, and pepper flakes. Mix well. Stir in the olives.

Toss the dressing with the oranges and serve.

YIELD: 4 SERVINGS

3 navel oranges

1 clove garlic, peeled and minced

2 tablespoons raw almond butter (see Note)

¼ teaspoon sea salt

¼ teaspoon hot pepper flakes (optional)

6 black olives, pitted and sliced

HEALTHFUL HINT: Oranges are a great source of bioflavonoids, which hasten the healing of athletic injury to joints. They are in short supply in orange juice, because bioflavonoids are concentrated in the membranes, pith, and central core. These are retained when the oranges are eaten whole.

NOTE: Raw almond butter is a nutritious alternative to mayonnaise, which contains sugars, refined oils and preservatives. It's rich in boron, which is important in maintaining joint health. Keep a jar on hand, in the refrigerator.

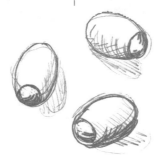

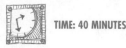

Parisian Steak Salad

Large slabs of meat draped across a dinner plate are "out". Smaller 3- to 4-ounce servings of meat are "in". This "light" steak dinner is an ideal way to enjoy a good piece of beef while also enjoying a variety of garden delights.

4 teaspoons Dijon mustard

12-ounces lean top round steak

½ cup purified water

¼ pound green beans, tips removed

2 scallions, trimmed and quartered

½ head romaine lettuce, torn, about 4 cups

8 cherry tomatoes

3 tablespoons balsamic vinegar

2 tablespoons extra virgin olive oil

1 teaspoon marjoram

¼ cup crumbled feta cheese (optional)

Position the oven rack about 3 inches from the broiler heat source. Preheat the broiler.

Spread 3 teaspoons of the mustard on both sides of the beef.

Broil the beef about 7 minutes on each side, for medium rare. Remove the steak from the broiler and allow it to cool for 5 minutes.

Place the water and green beans in a small saucepan, and steam, covered for 4 or 5 minutes, until bright green, yet still crispy. Pour the beans into a colander, run cold water over to stop the cooking, and let them drain.

Pulse chop the scallions. Combine them with the romaine, green beans, and tomatoes in a large bowl.

In a small bowl whisk together the vinegar, oil, marjoram, and the remaining 1 teaspoon mustard. Pour over greens and toss to combine. Using a sharp knife, slice the meat thinly across grain. Arrange the salad on individual servings plates. Top with beef slices, and sprinkle with feta cheese. Enjoy!

YIELD: 4 SERVINGS

Black-Eyed Pea Salad

This salad is terrific year-round, hot or cold, and it gets even better as it marinates. Use your favorite beans to keep changing this salad into a new recipe.

Lift beans out of the soaking water and into a medium-sized saucepan. Add fresh water and bay leaves.

Bring to a boil, partially covered, reduce flame, and simmer for 20 minutes.

Add ½ teaspoon salt and continue simmering for another 15 minutes (see Note).

Place a colander in a bowl and drain the beans. Put them in a medium bowl to cool slightly. Discard the bay leaves, and store cooking liquid for future use as a stock.

Pulse chop the onion, carrot, and parsley. Add to the beans with the Georgian Yogurt Sauce and stir. Allow the beans to marinate, unrefrigerated for 20 to 30 minutes, if time permits.

YIELD: 4 SERVINGS

Soak 1 cup sorted and washed black-eyed peas in purified water. (See page 198.)

2 cups soaked black-eyed peas (1 cup dry beans)

4 cups purified water

2 bay leaves

½ teaspoon sea salt

1 red onion, peeled and quartered

1 carrot, quartered

½ bunch parsley, thick stems removed

1 recipe Georgian Yogurt Sauce or other favorite dressing (page 67)

NOTE: Adding salt halfway through the cooking time keeps the beans from getting mushy and falling apart.

Herb 'n Onion Vinaigrette

Nothing beats the taste of homemade salad dressing, made with all quality ingredients such as the best olive oil and your favorite vinegars, herbs, and spices. Bottled dressings are full of sugar, salt, refined oils, chemicals, and preservatives—and those you can do without!

½ red, white, or yellow onion, peeled and cut in 2 pieces

1 clove garlic, peeled (optional)

¼ cup extra virgin olive oil

¼ cup flaxseed oil

¼ cup cider or balsamic vinegar

¼ cup lemon juice

2 teaspoons parsley or basil

½ teaspoon oregano or thyme

½ teaspoon herbal sea salt

Pinch ground pepper

In a blender, mince-chop the onion and garlic. Add the olive and flax oils, vinegar, lemon juice, parsley, oregano, herbal salt, and pepper. Puree until well blended.

Use on any salad greens, grains, or beans. Store in a covered jar, refrigerated. Can be stored for several weeks.

YIELD: 2 CUPS

HEALTHFUL HINT: Flaxseed oil is high in omega-3 essential fatty acids, the type that reduces inflammation and swelling. Canola oil has been promoted for its omega-3 content, which is much lower than flaxseed oil. It can be used in any recipe that calls for cold oil, since flaxseed oil should never be heated.

"A good cook is like a sorceress who dispenses happiness."

—Elsa Schiaparelli

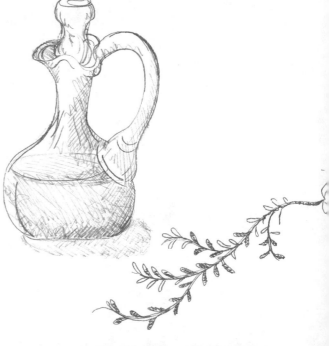

Garlic and Onion Dip

Here's a versatile dip that's a great mayonnaise replacer to spread on bread for a sandwich, pour on cooked potatoes or pasta for a salad, or thin and use as a creamy salad dressing. That is, of course, only if you can keep this dip around long enough—and not eat it all up with crackers, bread sticks, or chips!

Line a colander with paper toweling or coffee filters, or use a yogurt draining filter, placed in a bowl. Pour the yogurt in and set it aside for 30 minutes to drain the excess water.

Pour the drained yogurt into a medium mixing bowl. Add the garlic and onion flakes, parsley, oil, and salt. Stir to incorporate. Set aside for 10 minutes before serving.

Pour in a serving bowl and serve with bread sticks.

YIELD: 4 SERVINGS

HEALTHFUL HINT: Garlic and onions are known for their anti-inflammatory properties, and can be eaten at every meal. You can't get too much of these great arthritis fighters!

Drain 2 cups yogurt for 30 minutes before beginning recipe (see step 1).

2 cups plain yogurt with active cultures

1 tablespoon dried garlic flakes

1 tablespoon dried onion flakes

1 tablespoon dried parsley flakes, or 2 tablespoons chopped fresh parsley

1 tablespoon extra virgin olive oil

¼ teaspoon sea salt

Whole wheat sesame bread sticks

Perfect Party Dip with Raw Vegetable Spears

Here's a low calorie (about 20 calories per tablespoon) party dip with loads of flavor, which can easily be made from ingredients you already have at home!

1 cup plain yogurt with active cultures

2 tablespoons lemon juice or cider vinegar

2 tablespoons extra virgin olive oil or flaxseed oil

3 to 4 springs fresh parsley, thick stems removed

2 scallions, trimmed and coarsely chopped

½ teaspoon tarragon or basil

Pinch ground white pepper

A variety of vegetable spears, including carrots, celery, broccoli, scallions, jicama, or white radishes

P lace the yogurt, lemon juice, oil, parsley, scallions, tarragon or basil, and pepper in a blender or food processor. Blend together until mixture is smooth and creamy. With a rubber spatula, clean the sides of the container and blend again.

Pour dip into a ceramic bowl and place on a platter surrounded with the fresh vegetable spears.

YIELD: 4 SERVINGS

HEALTHFUL HINT: The raw vegetables in this dip have enzymes that help your body absorb all the good nutrients they contain to keep your bones and immune system strong.

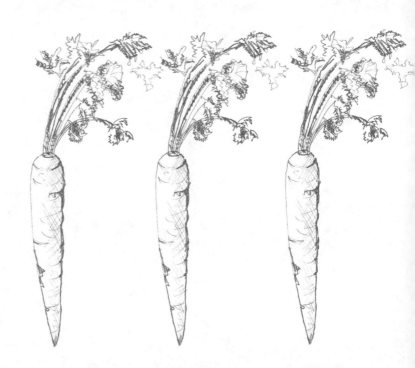

Lemon Almond-Mustard Dressing

Creamy, savory, and slightly tart, this dressing brings all of its best aspects to a salad. Pour it over red and green leaf lettuces, chicory, escarole, romaine, Boston, Bibb, radicchio, arugula, watercress, cabbage, Maché, or any other favorite salad.

Place the lemon juice, almond butter, 1/4 cup water, mustard, soy sauce, and salt in a blender. Blend well. Add additional water, if a thinner consistency is desired.

YIELD: 1 CUP

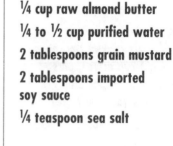

½ cup lemon juice

¼ cup raw almond butter

¼ to ½ cup purified water

2 tablespoons grain mustard

2 tablespoons imported soy sauce

¼ teaspoon sea salt

HEALTHFUL HINT: Almonds are rich in boron, which is important in maintaining joint health, and it helps to keep some bones from releasing free radicals. Boron can also be found in apples with their skins and in cauliflower.

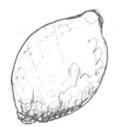

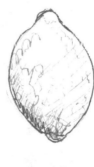

"You may have a fresh start any moment you choose, for this thing we call 'failure' is not the falling down, but the staying down."

—Mary Pickford

Hearty Hummus

Thankfully, hummus, a delicious Mid-Eastern dish is becoming an American staple. Most people enjoy it as a dip with pita bread or carrot and celery sticks. It can be used in place of heavy dressings on salads or as a spread in sandwiches.

Soak 1 cup of sorted and washed chickpeas (garbanzo beans) in purified water. Cook beans until soft. (See page 195)

2 ½ cups cooked chickpeas (from 1 cup dried), plus cooking liquid, or one 15-ounce jar (see Note)

2 to 3 cloves garlic, peeled

¼ cup lemon juice

¼ cup plain yogurt with active cultures

3 tablespoons sesame tahini

2 tablespoons extra virgin olive oil

½ to ¾ teaspoon sea salt

½ teaspoon ground cumin (optional)

NOTE: Some varieties of beans are now available in jars, and they taste much better than the canned ones —with no preservatives and less added salt. You can find them in a natural food store.

Drain the cooked chickpeas, reserving liquid. Using a blender or food processor, with the machine running, drop in the garlic, and chop finely.

Add the chickpeas and process until chickpeas are chopped and mealy.

Add the lemon juice, yogurt, tahini, oil, salt, and cumin. Process the mixture until smooth. From time to time, use a rubber spatula to scrape the sides of the processor bowl. If the puree seems dry, add a little of the bean cooking liquid. (Refrigerate the remaining liquid to use as a stock.)

Remove hummus to a serving bowl. Taste and adjust salt. (The salt and lemon in this recipe bring out the flavor of the garlic.)

YIELD: 3 CUPS

HEALTHFUL HINT: Prescription steroidal medicines taken to help osteoarthritis can cause the body to lose nutrients such as iron. Eating legumes such as chickpeas helps replenish lost iron.

Cilantro Salsa

Spoon this yummy salsa over beans and rice, scoop some up with corn chips, or pour it over chopped salad greens as a dressing.

In a blender or food processor, mince the cilantro. Remove it to a medium bowl. Mince both onions and add to the cilantro.

Stir in ½ cup water with the lime or lemon juice, oil, salt, and hot sauce. Stir and add more water as desired.

YIELD: 2 ¹/₂ CUPS

ALTHFUL HINT: Healthy food has eye appeal. These nutritious flavorings add color to e grains, beans, fish, or poultry — an attractive meal stimulates the appetite.

1 bunch cilantro, thick stems removed and washed

½ yellow or white onion, peeled and cut in half

½ red onion, peeled and cut in half

1 to 1½ cups purified water

¼ cup lime or lemon juice

2 tablespoons flaxseed oil or extra virgin olive oil

1 teaspoon sea salt

½ teaspoon hot sauce (optional)

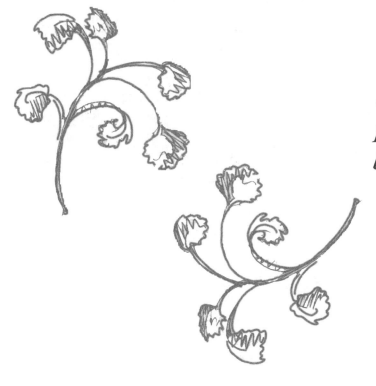

"Seeing is deceiving. It's eating that's believing."

—James Thurber

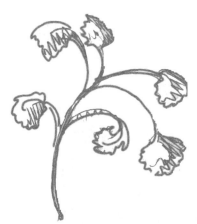

Tips for Dips

Here are some ideas to stimulate you to go beyond the same old chips for dips and salsas.

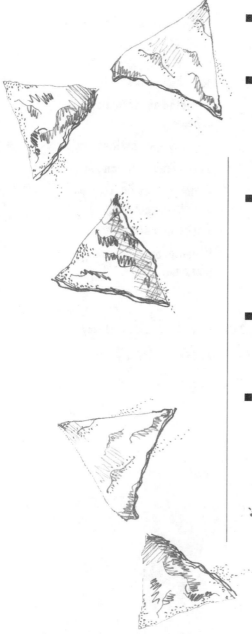

- **Pita Triangles** — Cut a whole grain pita bread in half, and each half into 3 or 4 pieces, creating triangles.

- **Pita Toast Points** — Slice a whole grain pita bread in half, creating 2 disks. Layer them on top of each other and cut into 6 or 8 pieces. Place them in the oven and bake at 350 degrees until golden and crisp. (Or toast whole grain bread slices, cut in quarters.)

- **Vegetable Spears, Medallions, and Slices** — Carrot spears, diakon radish medallions, celery sticks, scallion spears, cucumber rounds or spears, broccoli spears, cauliflower slices, jícama sticks, endive spears, fennel slices, and red, green, and yellow pepper slices.

- **Breads, Crackers, and Chips** — Rye crackers, whole grain bread cut in quarters, yellow and blue corn chips, whole grain baguette slices, and sesame whole wheat bread sticks.

- **Corn Tortillas** — Wrap some dip up in a tortilla for a quick and easy meal.

One-Pot Meals: Soups, Stews, and Stocks

Louisiana Gumbo with Okra

Yummy Red Lentil Soup

Purely Simple Egg Drop Soup

Latin Split Pea Soup with Chipotle Chile and Corn Chips

Yucatan Citrus Black Bean Soup

Winter Harvest Bisque with Toasted Almonds

French White Bean Cassoulet

Great Gazpacho

Lamb Stew with Leeks and Black Olives

Altogether Stew

Stocks: Beef, Chicken, Fish, and Vegetable

Louisiana Gumbo with Okra

This soup is more like a stew. It is a perfect dish to prepare when the family converges and is in need of some great homemade food. Serve with brown rice in the bottom of the bowl or on the side.

½ pound fresh okra, washed and trimmed

3 tablespoons unsalted butter or extra virgin olive oil

½ teaspoon ground black pepper

¼ teaspoon ground white pepper

¼ teaspoon cayenne powder

2 stalks celery, quartered

1 onion, peeled and quartered

½ green pepper, seeded and quartered

5 cups fish or chicken stock, homemade preferred, or purified water

1 ripe tomato, quartered

2 cloves garlic, peeled

½ teaspoon oregano or thyme

⅛ pound andouile or keilbasa sausage, cut into pieces, chemical-free preferred (optional)

½ pound raw medium shrimp, peeled and deveined

½ to 1 cup shucked oysters and juice

2 scallions, pulse chopped or sliced

½ to 1 teaspoon sea salt

2 teaspoons lemon juice

½ teaspoon filé or sassafras powder (optional)

Lemon wedges

Hot sauce

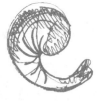

HEALTHFUL HINT: Okra is high in manganese, an important antioxidant that protects bone and cartilage formation. Others sources of this needed nutrient are nuts, seeds, whole grains, and leafy green vegetables.

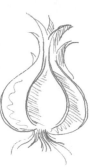

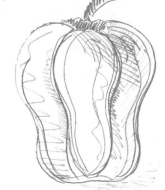

Remove and discard the okra stems. Using a blender or food processor, pulse chop the okra coarsely. Set ½ cup aside.

In a large stock pot, heat 2 tablespoons butter or oil and add all the okra except the ½ cup. Sauté on medium heat and add black and white peppers, and cayenne. Stir frequently, cooking until okra begins to brown, about 10 to 12 minutes.

Pulse chop the celery, onion, and green pepper. Add to the pot and continue sautéing for 5 more minutes. Stir occasionally, scraping the bottom of the pan.

Increase the heat, and add 1 cup stock. Cook uncovered, 5 minutes, stirring and scraping often.

Pulse chop the tomato and garlic, and add to the pot. Continue cooking, stirring frequently, another 5 minutes.

Add 2 more cups stock and continue cooking on a high flame, uncovered for 5 more minutes.

Add the remaining 1 tablespoon butter and 2 cups stock, and return to a boil. Add the oregano and sausage, and reduce heat. Simmer covered, for 45 minutes, stirring occasionally.

Add the remaining okra and cook 10 minutes.

Add the shrimp, oysters and juice, scallions, and salt. Stir and return to a boil, cooking for 1 or 2 more minutes, uncovered.

Add the lemon juice and give the gumbo one last stir.

Ladle gumbo into large bowls and sprinkle each with filé powder and serve with a lemon wedge. Offer a bottle of hot sauce, for those who like some additional heat!

YIELD: 4 TO 6 SERVINGS

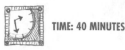

Yummy Red Lentil Soup

Those delicious lentil dishes found at Indian restaurants can easily be made at home—if you know the secret. And don't be surprised—when you cook red lentils, they change color—from pumpkin red to yellow ochre.

1 onion, peeled and quartered

2 cloves garlic, peeled

1 tablespoon unsalted butter

1 teaspoon curry powder or garam masala

1 teaspoon ground coriander

2 slices fresh ginger root

2 cups red lentils, sorted and washed

4 cups vegetable or chicken stock, homemade preferred, or purified water

3 tablespoons lemon juice

2 tablespoons extra virgin olive oil

1 teaspoon herbal sea salt

Several pinches ground pepper

¼ cup plain yogurt with active cultures

Using a blender or food processor, pulse chop the onion and garlic.

In a large soup pot, on medium heat, melt the butter and cook the onions until soft but not brown, about 5 minutes. Add the curry powder or garam masala, coriander, and ginger, and cook gently for another 30 seconds, being careful not to burn the spices.

Add the lentils and stock, and stir. Bring to a boil, covered. Lower heat and simmer, partially covered, until the lentils are tender, about 30 minutes, stirring occasionally.

Add the lemon juice, oil, salt, and pepper, and cook another minute. Remove ginger and discard.

Pour into individual bowls and serve with a dollop of yogurt, if desired.

Note: If red lentils are hard to find, substitute green or brown lentils or split peas, cooking them for 45 and 60 minutes, respectively.

YIELD: 4 TO 6 SERVINGS

HEALTHFUL HINT: Some people find beans difficult to digest. If this is the case for you, lentils are a good place to start, when you want more health-benefiting legumes in your diet. Lentils are high in protein and fiber, and many people find them easier to digest than other varieties of beans. The addition of curry spices and fresh ginger helps to aid in the digestion of beans, as well as giving a light and tasty flavor.

Purely Simple Egg Drop Soup

It's no wonder this wonderfully simple soup is a staple at most Chinese restaurants. A delightfully low-fat meal with a hint of essential protein, this soup is great when you want a tasty dish but don't have much time for cooking.

I n a medium-sized pot, on high heat, bring the stock to a boil, covered.

Add lemon juice and salt. Stir thoroughly.

Just before serving, drizzle the beaten egg into the simmering soup in a slow, steady stream, stirring constantly. When the egg coagulates, give the soup a stir. Ladle into bowls and serve topped with scallions.

YIELD: 4 TO 6 SERVINGS

3 ½ cups chicken stock, homemade preferred

1 teaspoon lemon juice (optional)

½ to 1 teaspoon herbal salt or sea salt

1 egg, organic preferred, slightly beaten

2 scallions, pulse chopped

ALTHFUL HINT: While a low-fat diet is optimal to keep the symptoms of arthritis at don't skimp on protein. Nature's finest protein creation is the egg, what scientists call a plete protein." The egg is a perfect combination of all the amino acids we need.

"Progress in civilization has been accompanied by progress in cookery."

—Fannie Farmer

Latin Split Pea Soup with Chipotle Chile and Corn Chips

Many people reminisce about a cup of Mom's homemade split pea soup, but this spicy version will warm your palate and your soul. It is bound to become a classic in your home. Mom might even ask for the recipe!

2 cups split peas, sorted and washed

1 ham bone, chemical-free preferred (optional)

4 cups chicken or vegetable stock, homemade preferred or purified water

1 bay leaf

1 teaspoon dried thyme

1 dry chipotle chile or 2 teaspoons chile powder

2 to 3 stalks celery, quartered

2 carrots, trimmed and quartered

2 cloves garlic, peeled

1 onion, peeled and quartered

1 to 1 ½ teaspoons sea salt

½ teaspoon ground pepper

1 tablespoon extra virgin olive oil or unsalted butter

Baked corn chips (see Note)

NOTE: If you cannot find baked chips, make your own by baking corn tortillas. Place them on a baking sheet, and bake at 325 degrees until crispy, about 15 minutes. Break them apart and serve!

In a large stock pot, over high heat, add the peas, ham bone, stock, bay leaf, and thyme. Bring to a boil, covered. Reduce heat to low, and cook until the peas begin to fall apart, about 60 minutes. Stir occasionally.

If using dried chipotle, soak it in water for 15 minutes. Remove the stem and seeds, and discard them along with the soaking water.

Using a blender or food processor, pulse mince the celery, carrots, garlic, onion, and chipotle.

Add the vegetables, salt, and pepper to the simmering soup. Cook another 15 minutes, covered, or until carrots are tender.

Using tongs, remove the ham bone and bay leaf. Add oil or butter. After cooling the bone, separate the meat and fat. Reserve meat. Discard the fat, bone, and bay leaf.

For a creamier soup, puree the soup in a blender or food processor, in small batches. As each batch is pureed, pour it into a soup tureen. Add the meat back to the soup, and stir well. Adjust consistency with additional stock or water, if a thinner soup is preferred.

Serve in a mug or bowl with a side of corn chips.

YIELD: 4 TO 6 SERVINGS

HEALTHFUL HINT: Most corn chips are fried in partially hydrogenated oils, which can induce and increase painful arthritic inflammation. We recommend the baked ones. Or you can make your own (see Note).

TIME: 1 HOUR

Yucatan Citrus Black Bean Soup

Forgot to soak the beans? Don't worry—this south-of-the border black bean staple can be made using a quick soaking method.

In a medium stock pot, on high heat, combine the soaked beans with the stock, bay leaf, oregano, cumin, and half the orange (¼). Bring to a boil, covered, reduce heat, and simmer until beans begin to soften, about 40 minutes.

Using a blender or food processor, pulse chop the onion, garlic, and tomato. Add to the beans with the salt, pepper, and oil. Cook until the beans are very tender, another 15 minutes.

Remove and discard the bay leaf. Puree the soup in the blender or food processor, in small batches, until the entire soup is smooth. Serve in individual bowls. Slice the remaining orange quarter and use as a garnish on the soup.

YIELD: 4 TO 6 SERVINGS

ALTHFUL HINT: If beans tend to give you gas, soak them for 6 to 8 hours, changing soaking water 2 or 3 times. Eating them more frequently will also help to alleviate this blem. (Or try a product called Beano®; see page 209.)

Soak 1 cup sorted and washed black beans in purified water (see page 195.)

2 cups soaked black beans (1 cup dry)

4 cups chicken or vegetable stock, homemade preferred, or purified water

1 bay leaf

¼ teaspoon oregano

⅛ teaspoon ground cumin

½ navel orange, unpeeled, organic preferred (see Note)

1 onion, peeled and quartered

1 clove garlic, peeled

1 ripe tomato, core removed and quartered

½ to 1 teaspoon sea salt

¼ teaspoon ground pepper

2 tablespoons extra virgin olive oil or unsalted butter

NOTE: When using the rind of any citrus, we suggest you use organic fruit, to avoid the many chemicals on the skin.

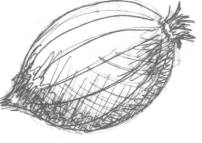

Winter Harvest Bisque with Toasted Almonds

Don't pass up this recipe because you think it is difficult to manage winter squash and yams. This soup is especially wonderful as summer turns into fall, and turning on the oven is a treat.

1 butternut, buttercup, or acorn squash, about 1 to 1 ½ pounds (see Note)

1 yam or sweet potato

½ cup almonds

1 onion, peeled and quartered

6 cups vegetable stock, homemade preferred or purified water

¾ teaspoon ground cinnamon

½ teaspoon ground ginger

½ teaspoon sea salt

2 tablespoons ghee or unsalted butter

2 tablespoons whole wheat flour

3 tablespoons lemon juice

¼ teaspoon ground white pepper

PREHEAT OVEN TO 450 DEGREES.

Place the whole squash and yam on a baking sheet. Bake the squash and yam until a fork easily pierces the vegetables, about 45 to 55 minutes. (The yam will cook faster and can be removed first.) Remove from the oven and cool. Cut the squash in half, remove the seeds and scoop the flesh out of the skin. Peel the yam and cut into large chunks. Set aside. Discard the skins.

Place the almonds in a cake pan or other small baking container, and bake alongside the squash and yam until golden and toasted, about 6 to 10 minutes. Stir the almonds after 4 or 5 minutes. Do not burn. Remove from the oven and pour into a bowl to cool.

Using a blender or food processor, pulse chop the onion to a coarse texture.

In a large stock pot, on a medium flame, heat the stock, and the add onion, squash, yam, cinnamon, ginger, and salt. Cover, and bring to a boil. Lower heat and simmer, about 15 to 20 minutes.

HEALTHFUL HINT: Cinnamon and ginger have long been used in herbal medicine to reduce inflammation. The beta-carotene in these orange starchy vegetables enhances immunity.

Prepare a roux by heating a skillet on a medium-high flame. Add the ghee or butter and flour. Stir constantly until fragrant, golden, and nutty-smelling, about 4 to 5 minutes. Take care that the roux does not smoke or burn.

Add 1/4 to 1/2 cup amounts of the stock mixture to the roux, continuing to stir and cook. Keep adding broth until the roux has the consistency of gravy. Pour into the stock pot and stir.

Add lemon juice, and pepper, and stir again.

In a blender or food processor, puree the soup in small batches, until the entire soup is smooth. Be careful when blending hot soup. Pour each batch into another pot or soup tureen. Once everything has been pureed, stir well.

Coarsely chop the toasted almonds. Ladle soup into bowls and top each with 1 tablespoon chopped almonds and serve.

YIELD: 2 1/2 QUARTS

NOTE: Avoid arduous chopping by baking or steaming hard vegetables first and then cutting them. Try this technique with carrots, turnips, rutabaga, beets, etc. In this recipe, the squash and yam can be baked ahead of time, or, if peeling and chopping don't present a problem for you, peel them and cut them into large chunks and proceed.

French White Bean Cassoulet

As satisfying and fragrant a pot of beans as you're likely to make. Any leftover can be turned into a bountiful soup with some additional water or stock!

Soak 1 cup of sorted and washed white beans in water (see page 195)

2 cups soaked white beans (1 cup dry) (see Note 1)

3 to 4 cups salt-free stock, or purified water (see Note 2)

Pinch rosemary

1 bay leaf

1 onion, peeled and quartered

4 cloves garlic, peeled

2 tomatoes, quartered

4 tablespoons unsalted butter or extra virgin olive oil

2 carrots, trimmed and quartered

1 parsnip, trimmed and quartered

1 teaspoon herbal sea salt

¼ teaspoon ground white pepper

½ cup whole grain bread crumbs or ground sunflower seeds

¼ cup chopped parsley

½ teaspoon thyme

¼ teaspoon marjoram

¼ teaspoon sea salt

Drain the beans and place in a large, ovenproof Dutch oven. Add 2 ½ cups stock, rosemary, and bay leaf. Bring to a boil, covered, over medium heat and cook until the beans are soft, about 45 minutes. Add additional stock, as necessary.

In a blender or food processor, pulse chop the onion, garlic, and tomatoes. In a separate pot or skillet, heat 2 tablespoons butter and add the chopped vegetables. Cover and cook on medium heat until softened, about 15 minutes, stirring occasionally.

Pulse chop or cut the carrots and parsnip, and add to the onion mixture with ½ cup stock. Cover and continue cooking another 20 minutes. Stir occasionally.

Preheat the oven to 350 degrees.

HEALTHFUL HINT: Beans are a good source of iron and potassium, both of which counter the use of NSAIDs, steroids and other medications. They also offer quality protein which is free of arachodonic acid, an inflammation producer.

NOTE 1: Leftover cooked beans can be used, which will reduce the cooking and preparation time for this recipe by 1 hour. There are many varieties of white beans, including Great Northern, lima, navy, and cannellini.

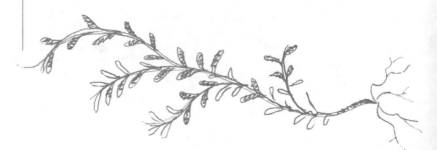

Season the beans with remaining 2 tablespoons butter, herbal salt, and pepper, stirring well. The beans should be moist and soupy. Add additional stock, if needed. Remove half of the beans to a separate bowl. Place the cooked tomato mixture in an even layer on top of the beans remaining in the pot. Layer the remaining beans on top of the vegetables.

In a small bowl, mix the bread crumbs, parsley, thyme, marjoram, and sea salt. Top the beans with the crumb mixture. Bake uncovered about 30 to 40 minutes or until beans are quite tender.

YIELD: 4 TO 6 SERVINGS

NOTE 2: To soften beans, they need to be cooked in a salt-free liquid. The salt is added after.

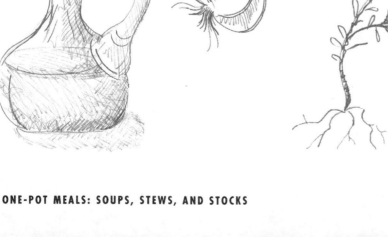

Great Gazpacho

A good gazpacho recipe is like an heirloom—most families pass it down from generation to generation. This recipe, in particular, is so surprisingly tasty—and easy to prepare—that you won't believe how good it is for you!

1 or 2 cloves garlic, peeled

½ small onion, red preferred, peeled

1 ½ pounds ripe beefsteak or plum tomatoes, quartered (about 4 cups) (see Note)

2 slices whole grain bread, broken into pieces

1 ½ cups purified water

1 teaspoon sea salt

3 tablespoons extra virgin olive oil

3 tablespoons cider or wine vinegar

¼ teaspoon hot pepper sauce (optional)

¼ cup plain yogurt with active cultures

GARNISHES: chopped red or green pepper, diced cucumber, sliced scallion, whole grain croutons

In a blender or processor, pulse chop the garlic, onion, and tomatoes. Pour into a large bowl.

Add the bread, ½ cup water, salt, oil, vinegar, and pepper sauce. Toss once, cover, and refrigerate. Marinate about 30 minutes.

Put the marinated ingredients in a blender or processor, and puree until the tomato and bread is completely smooth.

Stir in the remaining 1 cup water. Add additional water, if a thinner consistency is desired.

Chill until very cold before serving. Either fill a bowl with ice and wedge a second bowl into the ice and pour the soup in to cool, or refrigerate, stirring occasionally. Taste and adjust seasonings.

Pour gazpacho into a bowl and swirl several tablespoons of yogurt around the edge. Garnish with any or all of the suggested condiments.

YIELD: 4 TO 6 SERVINGS

NOTE: For the best taste, it is very important to choose very ripe and slightly soft tomatoes. The beefsteak tomatoes will be juicier than the plum, but they can both be used with equal success. Vine ripened tomatoes are at their height at the middle to the end of the summer, and will yield the best tasting soup. Also, don't store tomatoes in the refrigerator. They lose flavor quite rapidly when cold.

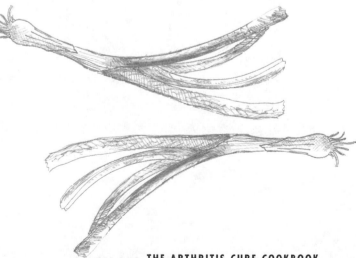

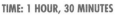

TIME: 1 HOUR, 30 MINUTES

Lamb Stew with Leeks and Black Olives

These luscious flavors will melt in your mouth, full of the sweetness of onions and carrots, the aroma of black olives, and the subtle intensity of mustard and tomatoes.

Place the flour in a wide bowl and add the lamb, tossing in the flour to coat. Heat a large casserole, and add 2 tablespoons ghee. Add a few lamb cubes at a time and cook until browned on all sides. Do not crowd the pan. Remove the browned lamb to a plate or bowl and continue cooking the lamb cubes until golden brown.

Add the remaining ghee and flour to the casserole, along with the leeks. Stir and cook on medium heat.

In a blender or food processor, pulse chop the carrots and garlic. Add to the leek mixture along with the thyme, stir well and continue cooking until carrots are soft, about 15 minutes.

Pulse chop the tomato. Add the stock and lamb. Stir, scraping the bottom to loosen any browned particles. Cover and simmer gently, stirring occasionally until the lamb is tender, about 45 minutes.

Add the potatoes, cover and cook until soft, about another 20 minutes.

In a small bowl, add ¼ cup of the liquid from the stew and dilute the mustard in it. Season with salt and pepper, and return mixture to the stew, mixing well. Add the olives and cook covered, another 5 minutes.

Stir 3 tablespoons of parsley into the stew. Spoon into a large serving bowl. Sprinkle the remaining parsley on top, and serve.

YIELD: 4 TO 6 SERVINGS

¼ cup whole grain flour seasoned with sea salt and ground pepper

2 pounds lamb stewing meat, cut into 1½-inch chunks

½ cup ghee, unsalted butter, or extra virgin olive oil

4 leeks, cleaned and cut into 2-inch pieces

2 carrots, trimmed and quartered

2 cloves garlic, peeled

1 teaspoon dried thyme

1 tomato, quartered

3 cups beef or vegetable stock, homemade preferred

3 potatoes, peeled and quartered

1 tablespoon prepared grain mustard

1 teaspoon sea salt

½ teaspoon ground pepper

¼ cup oil-cured black or Greek olives

4 tablespoons chopped parsley

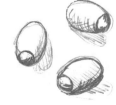

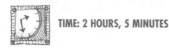

Altogether Stew

A meal in one pot, this stew combines the best of everything—beans, grains, and poultry. Make a batch on the weekend, and you'll have meals all week. This stew simmers for hours, and uses large chunks of vegetables to cut down on chopping time.

Soak ½ cup sorted and washed chick peas in purified water (see page 195.)

1 cup soaked chickpeas (½ cup dry)

4 cups purified water or any stock except fish

1 bay leaf

1 pound deboned chicken or turkey, cut into pieces

2 tablespoons whole grain flour

1½ teaspoons herbal sea salt

1 teaspoon oregano

1 teaspoon basil

¼ teaspoon red pepper flakes

8 button mushrooms

4 cloves garlic, peeled

2 carrots, trimmed and quartered

2 potatoes, peeled and quartered

2 stalks celery, quartered

1 onion, peeled and quartered

1 sweet red pepper, seeded and cut into 8 pieces

½ butternut squash or sweet potato, peeled and cut into 2-inch cubes

1 cup whole grain couscous, bulgur, or orzo

4 sprigs parsley, leaves only

Place the soaked peas in a large Dutch oven. Add the water or stock and bay leaf. Bring to a boil, covered, lower flame, and simmer 1 hour (see Note).

Add the chicken and sprinkle with flour, salt, oregano, basil, and pepper flakes. Stir well. Add the mushrooms, garlic, carrots, potatoes, celery, onion, sweet pepper, and squash. Stir again, cover and cook 45 minutes.

Push the stew toward the sides of the pot, making a well in the center. Add the couscous to the liquid and stir. Cover and cook until the couscous swells, about 10 minutes. Add additional liquid, if needed.

Spoon onto a large platter and garnish with parsley leaves.

YIELD: 4 TO 6 SERVINGS

HEALTHFUL HINT: Don't use dull knives when cutting. It takes more muscle power and unnecessarily strains the joints. Use a blender, food processor or a mini-chopper to ease your efforts.

NOTE: Leftover cooked beans can be used in this recipe, which will reduce the cooking and preparation time by 1 hour.

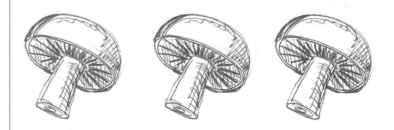

Stocks: Beef, Chicken, Fish, and Vegetable

Basic stocks are easy to make, take very little effort, and are a great way to include flavor-rich nutrients in your foods. Poultry, beef, and vegetables can be used to make rich tasting liquids which can replace water in any recipe. Sometimes lentils or other beans are added to give a vegetarian stock a more robust and "meaty" flavor. Most stocks can be used interchangeably in recipes, except for fish stock, although a fish recipe that calls for stock can be substituted with a poultry or vegetable stock.

Wash the bones and/or peelings and place them in a large stock pot with the water, bay leaf, and vinegar. Add any of the desired flavor enhancers and make sure the water covers the ingredients by 1-inch. Cover and bring to a boil.

Reduce flame and simmer until the meat falls off the bones, or the fish head falls apart, about 1½ hours. Cook vegetable stocks until the vegetables are soft, about 50 to 60 minutes, or 40 minutes if using peelings.

Place a colander in a large bowl, and carefully strain the stock. Discard the bones, vegetables, and spices.

Use the stock right away or set it aside to cool. Once cooled, pour the stock into storage containers. Indicate the type of stock and date on each container, and refrigerate or freeze them. Stock will last for 7 to 10 days refrigerated or up to 6 months frozen.

NOTE:

For Beef Stock: Include bones such as shanks, neck, knuckle, leg, and/or oxtails. If the bones are very large, ask your butcher to cut them. This to allow more surface

1 to 3 pounds raw beef bones; or poultry bones, feet, and/or innards; or fish bones and head (white meat only); or 6 to 8 cups of vegetables and/or vegetable peelings (see Note)

4- to 5-quarts water

1 bay leaf

1 or 2 teaspoons cider vinegar

EALTHFUL HINT: Seasonings such as tomatoes and vinegar add a spark of flavor and ˙aw out minerals from the bones and peelings. Using stock in recipes, is an easy way to incor-˙rate additional nutrients in your meals.

To these ingredients, add any or all of the following flavor enhancers;

3 to 4 sprigs parsley

3 or 4 black or white pepper corns

3 to 6 coriander seeds

2 chopped tomatoes

1 onion, quartered (peeling is not necessary)

1 carrot, quartered

½ orange or lemon peel, organic preferred

¼ cup green lentils, sorted and washed

area to be exposed and more flavor and nutrients will be released.

For Poultry Stock: Use chicken, turkey or duck bones such as backs, necks, feet, and/or gizzards. Do not use the livers. A whole chicken can be boiled in water and the meat used as is, in salad, or sliced for sandwiches, saving the stock for later use.

For Fish Stock: Only use white meat fish such as cod, scrod, red snapper, catfish, flounder, or sole. Use the bones, tail, fins, and head.

For Vegetable Stock: Any combination of vegetables including onions, garlic, leeks, carrots, parsnips, parsley root, celery stalks with leaves, celeriac (celery root), or butternut, acorn, or buttercup squash, cut into large pieces. Also, use vegetable peelings such as onion and garlic skins, corn cobs, winter squash seeds, and all types of potato skins. The stock will be sweeter tasting if the peelings are from organic vegetables. Do not include cruciferous vegetables when making stock, such as cabbage, broccoli, cauliflower, and brussels sprouts, they are strong tasting and can be over powering.

YIELD: ABOUT 4-QUARTS

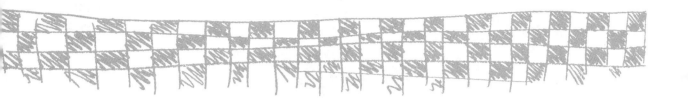

Vegetables

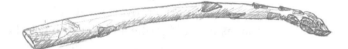

Kale with Capers and Pine Nuts

Baked Yam Rounds with Cinnamon Butter

Curried Cauliflower with Cashews

Garden Fresh Rosemary Green Beans

Mexican Succotash

Italian Baked Asparagus

Mushroom Tapenade

Golden Crowned Tomatoes

Kale with Capers and Pine Nuts

These hearty leafy greens are a great way to increase your intake of fiber and minerals. Leftover, they are remarkable stuffed into a pita bread or tossed into a bean soup.

6 cups purified water

1 bunch kale (see Note)

3 tablespoons extra virgin olive oil

4 cloves garlic, peeled and sliced or cut in half

2 tablespoons pine nuts

Large pinch nutmeg

Pinch sea salt

1 tablespoon capers

Juice of 1 lemon

NOTE: Any dark leafy greens will make a fine substitute for kale. Try collards, broccoli rabe, mustard or turnip greens, or dandelions. Swiss chard and spinach are cooked by another method and will not stand up well to the long boiling process.

In a large stock pot, bring water to a boil, covered. Place the kale in boiling water, return pot to a boil, uncovered, and cook, until tender, about 10 minutes.

Drain, reserving broth as desired.

In a large skillet, over a medium flame, heat 2 tablespoons oil. Add garlic and pine nuts, and cook until the nuts just begin to toast and the garlic browns on the edges, 4 to 5 minutes.

Pulse or hand chop the greens coarsely and add to the pan. Add nutmeg and salt. Cook another 5 minutes, uncovered, stirring frequently.

Add the capers, lemon juice, and remaining 1 tablespoon oil. Toss well and cook for another minute. Place seasoned greens in a bowl. Serve warm or at room temperature.

YIELD: 4 SERVINGS

HEALTHFUL HINT: Greens are full of alpha-linolenic acid (ALA), which is an omega-3 fatty acid, the one that blocks the production of overzealous prostaglandins and leukotrienes. ALA is essential as an inflammation fighter. The cooking liquid from these greens has a high level of these and many other useful minerals, so pour some into a mug and add a little lemon or herbal salt. Enjoy this warm nutritious broth while you finish cooking your meal.

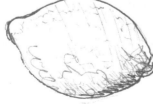
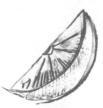

Baked Yam Rounds with Cinnamon Butter

Keep cooked yams on hand in order to prepare this dish in minutes. Served hot or at room temperature, this recipe satisfies any sweet tooth, with very few calories.

PREHEAT OVEN TO 450 DEGREES.

Place the yams or sweet potatoes on a baking pan and place in the oven until soft when pierced with a fork, about 45 minutes.

Remove yams from the oven, and using a fork and a knife, without peeling, carefully cut each yam in 3 or 4 round pieces. Smear each round with a little butter on both sides. Sprinkle with cinnamon and a tiny bit of salt.

Place under the broiler for 3 or 4 minutes, until bubbly and golden brown. Using a spatula, place yams on a serving platter, golden side up.

YIELD: 4 SERVINGS

3 yams or sweet potatoes unpeeled, scrubbed

3 tablespoons unsalted butter, room temperature

1 teaspoon cinnamon

Pinch sea salt

HEALTHFUL HINT: These deep orange spuds are a bonus for arthritis patients because they are extremely high in vitamin A, which fortifies the immune system.

Curried Cauliflower with Cashews

This delicious recipe is the perfect accompaniment for fish or chicken dishes, and a pleasing addition to a vegetarian entree.

2 teaspoons unsalted butter

1 teaspoon curry powder

¼ cup whole raw cashews

½ to ¾ cup purified water

½ teaspoon sea salt

1 head cauliflower, broken into florets

1 tablespoon flax seed oil or unsalted butter

Melt the butter in a large skillet, over medium heat. Add the curry powder and cashews, and cook until nuts are toasted and golden, about 3 minutes, stirring frequently. Transfer nuts to a large serving bowl.

Add the water and salt to the skillet, and bring to a boil. Add the cauliflower, lower flame and cover. Steam 10 minutes.

Add the cauliflower to the serving bowl. Drizzle with flax seed oil, and toss with the cashews. Serve warm.

YIELD: 4 SERVINGS

HEALTHFUL HINT: Cauliflower contains boron, a mineral that in studies has been shown to have a beneficial effect on osteoarthritis. We used flax seed oil for a rich garnish because like fish oils, flax oil lowers arthritic inflammation (and cholesterol).

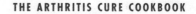

Garden Fresh Rosemary Green Beans

Take garden-fresh beans and turn them into a gourmet dish that is rich and satisfying—but low in fat.

In a 2-quart saucepan, steam the green beans in water for 5 minutes, covered. Drain and remove beans to a serving bowl or platter. Reserve the liquid in a small bowl.

In a blender or food processor, pulse chop the onion and garlic. Add the oil, onion, garlic, and rosemary to the saucepan. Sauté until the onion becomes translucent, about 3 minutes. Stir in the flour and cook the mixture for 1 more minute. Stir in the reserved cooking liquid and continue cooking constantly, stirring until slightly thickened. Add additional water as needed.

Add the green beans and mix well. Cook over medium heat, uncovered, until the beans are heated through, about 2 minutes.

YIELD: 4 SERVINGS

½ pound green beans, trimmed

½ cup purified water

1 onion, peeled and quartered

2 cloves garlic, peeled

2 teaspoons extra virgin olive oil

1 teaspoon rosemary

1 tablespoon whole wheat flour

HEALTHFUL HINT: Green vegetables such as these green beans contain alpha-linoleic acid, one of the essential oils that keep joints well lubricated.

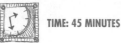
Mexican Succotash

Enjoy this dish in the summer when you can find these ingredients at their freshest and most nutritious. Experiment with different combinations of vegetables, and you'll combine a range of nutrients.

1 onion, peeled and quartered

2 tablespoons unsalted butter

1 or 2 zucchini, or ¼ pound green beans

1 cup corn kernels, fresh (cut from 1 or 2 ears) (see Note)

1 teaspoon thyme

¼ teaspoon herbal sea salt

¼ teaspoon ground black pepper

NOTE: To make cutting the kernels off the cob easier, break the corn in half.

Using a blender or food processor, pulse mince the onion. Melt the butter in a large skillet on a medium-high flame. Add the onion and sauté until soft, about 5 minutes.

Pulse chop the zucchini or green beans and add to the onions along with the corn, thyme, herbal salt, and pepper; toss the ingredients lightly. Cover the skillet, and cook over low heat for 15 minutes, stirring occasionally.

YIELD: 4 SERVINGS

HEALTHFUL HINT: If you really love corn and cannot manage to cut the kernels off the cob, this is a recipe in which frozen corn would be acceptable. To give yourself the best, purchase frozen organic corn kernels from your natural food store.

> *"In Des Moines, a man's eyes will light up at the mere mention of the word 'corn.'"*
>
> —Philip Hamburger

Italian Baked Asparagus

Everyone loves asparagus. What makes this recipe truly special is that you can prepare it from items generally found in your kitchen, so the prospect of a tasty meal is never far away.

PREHEAT OVEN TO 425 DEGREES.

Place the asparagus and water in a shallow baking pan. Drizzle oil over them.

Using a blender or food processor, pulse chop the garlic and parsley. Sprinkle over the asparagus, along with the salt and pepper.

Bake uncovered, until tender but firm to the touch, about 10 to 15 minutes.

YIELD: 4 SERVINGS

1 pound asparagus, tough ends removed

½ cup purified water

2 tablespoons extra virgin olive oil

2 cloves garlic, peeled

2 sprigs Italian parsley, thick stems removed and washed

Sea salt

Ground black pepper

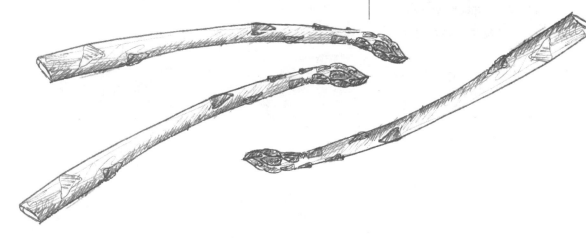

Mushroom Tapenade

Enjoy this unique recipe alongside an entree, or with a salad and bread for a simple meal. It has the feeling of extravagance and the taste to match!

1 package dried bolete mushrooms (¾ ounce) (see Note)

Purified water

One 8- to 10-ounce carton white button mushrooms

2 tablespoons extra virgin olive oil

1 tablespoon unsalted butter

2 sprigs Italian parsley, thick stems removed and washed

1 clove garlic, peeled

¼ to ½ teaspoon sea salt

¼ teaspoon ground pepper

NOTE: Bolete mushrooms refers to varieties such as cèpes and porcini. If they are available fresh, substitute ¼ pound for the dried measure. Shiitake, oyster, cremini, or chanterelles can also be substituted.

In a small bowl, soak bolete mushrooms in plenty of water until soft, about 15 minutes. Remove mushrooms and squeeze slightly to release excess water, and pulse chop or slice.

In a blender or food processor, slice or pulse chop the button mushrooms.

In a medium skillet, heat the oil and butter, and add all the mushrooms. Cook uncovered, over moderate heat, stirring often. Allow the edges of the mushrooms to begin to brown.

Pulse chop the parsley and garlic. Add to the mushrooms, and season with salt and pepper. Cook 2 or 3 minutes more, stirring occasionally. Serve hot, or at room temperature.

YIELD: 4 SERVINGS

HEALTHFUL HINT: Corticosteroids can increase appetite, so it's a good idea to make low calorie gourmet foods such as these mushrooms a staple on your shopping list. They are also a good source of potassium, a mineral easily excreted when taking some arthritis medications

Golden Crowned Tomatoes

This easy to make and terrific tomato dish is too good to pass up when tomatoes are at their peak. Share them with your family as a perky vegetable dish along side chops or at room temperature with Quick and Easy Chinese Chicken Salad (page 70).

PREHEAT OVEN TO 375 DEGREES.

Grease a baking pan with 1 teaspoon oil. Place the 4 tomato halves on the pan, open side up, and bake for 5 minutes.

In a blender or food processor, pulse chop the parsley and garlic. Put them in a small bowl and add the bread crumbs, sunflower seeds, herbal salt, and pepper.

Spoon the bread crumb mixture onto tomato tops and bake until the tops are golden, about another 10 minutes. Serve hot or at room temperature.

YIELD: 4 SERVINGS

HEALTHFUL HINT: Some people find certain foods such as wheat, dairy products, tomatoes, and peppers to have an inflaming and painful effect. Keep track of symptoms after eating certain foods. You are your own best authority on how you feel.

3 tablespoons extra virgin olive oil

2 large tomatoes, halved horizontally

2 sprigs parsley, thick stems removed and washed

1 clove garlic, peeled

1 cup whole grain bread crumbs

¼ cup raw sunflower seeds

½ teaspoon herbal sea salt

¼ teaspoon ground pepper

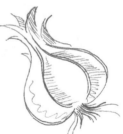

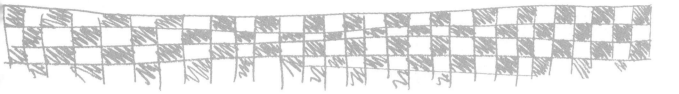

Vegetarian Entrees

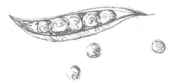

Lasagna alla Pesto

California-Style Broccoli Rabe, Roasted Garlic, and Portobello Focaccia

Eternal Life Seven Vegetable Stew

Gourmet Leek-Onion Quiche

Moroccan Tagine with Savory Saffron Couscous

Enchiladas Squared

Texas-Inspired Chili

Indian-Style Curried Eggs

French Red Lentil Pâté

Lasagna alla Pesto

We've cut out the pasta cooking step—a real time saver—so this can become an easy-to-make holiday favorite. Our version of lasagna finds its rich health benefits from layers of spinach.

1 pound fresh spinach, thick stems removed and washed

1 ¾ cups purified water

1 onion, peeled and quartered

3 tablespoons extra virgin olive oil

¼ teaspoon sea salt

⅛ teaspoon ground pepper

1 pound mozzarella cheese, organic preferred

4 cups (2 pounds) ricotta cheese, organic preferred

½ cup grated Parmesan cheese, organic preferred

One 8-ounce box whole wheat lasagna noodles, uncooked

1 recipe Perfect Pesto (see page 163)

Place spinach and ½ cup water in a medium skillet. Bring to a boil, covered, lower flame, and steam until spinach has wilted, about 4 minutes. Drain and allow to cool. Rinse skillet.

In a blender or food processor, pulse chop the onion. Add to the skillet with 2 tablespoons oil, and sauté the onion until soft, about 5 minutes. Season with salt and pepper. Turn off heat and set aside.

Pulse chop mozzarella or grate it on the coarse side of a cheese grater.

Squeeze or press the juice out of spinach. Coarsely pulse or hand chop and combine in a large bowl with the onion, ricotta, and Parmesan. Mix well. In a small bowl, add 1 cup water to Perfect Pesto and stir to blend.

PREHEAT OVEN TO 350 DEGREES.

Grease a deep 9- x 13-inch baking pan with the remaining 1 tablespoon oil. Pour ¼ cup water into the pan. Place a layer of uncooked lasagna noodles in the pan.

HEALTHFUL HINT: Dark-green vegetables such as spinach are filled with carotenoid compounds, vitamins E and B6, bioflavonoids, iron, and magnesium, all of which are good to heal arthritis.

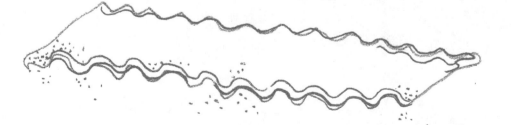

Spread one-third of the spinach filling onto the noodles. Pour 1 cup Perfect Pesto and water mixture evenly over noodles; sprinkle with one-quarter of the mozzarella mixture. Add another layer of pasta, and repeat the procedure. Top with one final layer of noodles and the remaining pesto sauce. Sprinkle with remaining mozzarella (see Note).

Cover with parchment paper, then foil, and bake for 45 to 50 minutes. Remove the covering, and brown the top, baking another 5 to 10 minutes.

Remove from the oven. Loosely place parchment paper over top and allow lasagna to sit for 5 to 10 minutes before serving. Cut into large squares and serve with a salad.

YIELD: 6 TO 8 SERVINGS (IMPOSSIBLE TO MAKE LESS — BUT LEFTOVERS FREEZE WELL!)

NOTE: Assemble lasagna ahead of time and bake it later, or pre-bake this dish and reheat it at the time of serving.

California-Style Broccoli Rabe, Roasted Garlic, and Portobello Focaccia

Don't feel like you have to deprive yourself of delicious dishes such as pizza, and focaccia. This version is not only tasty, but is also full of healthy ingredients. A great way to include mineral-rich greens!

4 tablespoons extra virgin olive oil

2 heads garlic, peeled (about 20 cloves)

1 small bunch broccoli rabe, thick stems removed (see Note)

1 portobello mushroom cap, quartered, or ¼ pound button mushrooms

Dash of dried red pepper flakes (optional)

Pinch sea salt

One 12-inch whole grain prepared crust (such as Za-Pit-za), or 6 slices whole grain Italian bread

2 ounces feta or goat cheese

½ teaspoon oregano or basil

NOTE: Any dark leafy greens such as collards and kale can be used in this recipe. Since the leaves are so large, chop or tear each leaf in 3 or 4 pieces before cooking.

In a large skillet, on medium flame, heat 2 tablespoons oil and cook the whole garlic cloves until lightly browned, about 10 to 12 minutes. Remove to a small bowl.

Add another tablespoon of oil to the skillet along with the broccoli rabe, and cook on a medium-low flame, until wilted, about 3 minutes. Pulse chop or slice mushroom, and add with the pepper flakes to the skillet. Cook on medium heat, covered, stirring often, until the broccoli rabe is tender and the mushroom is soft. Turn heat off and uncover.

PREHEAT OVEN TO 425 DEGREES.

Place the dough or bread on a pizza stone or baking pan, and drizzle with remaining oil. Spoon on the greens mixture, and distribute the garlic cloves evenly over the top. Crumble the cheese on top and sprinkle with oregano or basil.

Bake until the crust is browned and crisp, and the topping is piping hot, about 15 to 25 minutes. (Baking time will vary if using pre-baked bread; start to check after 10 minutes, and check frequently after that.) Over-baking will harden the crust.

YIELD: 4 TO 6 SERVINGS

HEALTHFUL HINT: Focaccia and pizza can be healthy when made this way. Incorporating a dark-leafy green, such as broccoli rabe, is a great way to consume beta carotene, one of the many carotenoids.

Eternal Life Seven Vegetable Stew

Conceived on the banks of Banaras, the "eternal city" in India, this hearty dish will give you a day's allowance of vegetables—and a delicious meal at the same time. Serve on whole grain basmati rice or udon noodles. Scoop some leftovers on top of toast for a great lunch.

In a blender or food processor, pulse chop garlic and ginger finely.

Heat the butter in a large pot, on a high flame. Add the garlic and ginger, and sauté until golden, about 1 minute.

Add the cumin, coriander, and turmeric, and turn off the flame. Stir thoroughly.

Pulse chop the tomatoes. Add ¼ cup cashews and tahini, and puree until smooth. Add ½ cup water and salt, and puree again. Pour into the pot with the remaining 1 cup water, and bring to a boil on a medium-high flame, covered. Reduce heat and simmer, about 8 minutes.

Add the onion, potatoes, cauliflower, eggplant, kohlrabi or turnip, and bell pepper. Continue simmering, covered, until the vegetables are tender, about 25 minutes.

Pulse chop fresh coriander and add along with peas to stew. Stir to incorporate and cook for another 1 or 2 minutes, covered.

Taste and add salt, if needed. Spoon stew into a large tureen or bowl, and garnish with the remaining ¼ cup cashews.

YIELD: 4 SERVINGS

3 garlic cloves, peeled

1 walnut-sized knob fresh ginger root

2 tablespoons unsalted butter, ghee or extra virgin olive oil

1 ½ teaspoons ground cumin

½ teaspoon ground coriander

¼ teaspoon ground turmeric

5 plum tomatoes, quartered

½ cup raw cashews, unsalted

1 tablespoon sesame tahini paste

1 ½ cups purified water

½ teaspoon sea salt, or to taste

4 small white onions, peeled and left whole

6 small red, white, or Yukon gold potatoes, about 2 inches in diameter

½ head cauliflower, broken into florets

1 small eggplant, trimmed, unpeeled, cut into cubes

2 kohlrabi or white turnips, trimmed and quartered

1 large, sweet, red bell pepper, seeds and inner ribs removed, coarsely pulse chopped

4 stems fresh coriander (see Note)

½ cup fresh peas, sugar snaps, or snow peas

NOTE: Fresh coriander is also called Chinese parsley or cilantro.

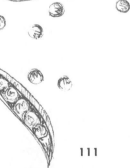

HEALTHFUL HINT: Include ginger in foods frequently. It will help to reduce swelling and to override the discomforts from inflammatory osteoarthritis.

Gourmet Leek-Onion Quiche

This light quiche conjures up memories of quaint Parisian cafes. You can have the same dining experience right at home, providing all the best nutrients for your body, mind, and soul.

2 white or yellow onions, peeled and quartered

1 red onion, peeled and quartered

2 tablespoons extra virgin olive oil

2 leeks, whites and 2 inches of green parts only, timmed and well rinsed

1 tablespoon fresh tarragon or thyme, or 1 teaspoon dried

½ teaspoon herbal sea salt

¼ teaspoon ground black pepper

¼ cup purified water

3 eggs, organic preferred

¼ cup plain yogurt or butter-milk with active cultures

1 prepared whole wheat pie crust (see Note)

Grated Parmesan or Romano cheese, organic preferred (optional)

NOTE: Whole wheat pie crusts are available in the frozen section at the natural food store. If this isn't available, make a crust-less quiche, by buttering the pie pan and sprinkling it with whole grain bread crumbs. Pour the filling in and bake as usual.

In a blender or food processor, pulse chop the white, yellow, and red onions. Remove to a bowl.

Heat the oil in a large skillet, on a medium-high flame. Sauté the onions until richly browned and caramelized, about 12 to 15 minutes, stirring often. Adjust heat as necessary to prevent burning.

Pulse chop the leeks and tarragon. Add to the skillet with the salt and pepper. Stir well. Add the water and cover, cooking until leeks are soft, another 7 to 10 minutes.

Transfer the onion mixture to a large platter or bowl and cool completely.

PREHEAT OVEN TO 425 DEGREES.

In a blender or medium bowl, whisk the eggs and yogurt or buttermilk together.

Arrange leek-onion mixture in a thick layer over the pie crust. Pour the egg mixture over all.

Bake for 10 minutes. Lower heat to 350 degrees and bake for another 30 to 35 minutes, or until the eggs are set and the crust is golden brown. If using cheese, sprinkle some over the top during the last 10 minutes of baking, allowing it to melt.

Allow quiche to cool about 5 minutes, to set. Cut into wedges and serve.

YIELD: 4 SERVINGS

HEALTHFUL HINT: Onions supply antioxidants, which neutralize free-radicals, the joint busters.

Moroccan Tagine with Savory Saffron Couscous

Take a mental trip to Marakesh as you prepare this stew with its abundance of aromatic flavors.

In a large pot, combine the lentils and stock. Bring to a boil, covered, lower heat, and simmer for 35 minutes.

In a blender or food processor, pulse chop the garlic, carrot, yam, and onion, (if using pearl onions, don't pulse chop). Add vegetables to the lentils with the lemon juice, and spices. Cook covered, until the beans are soft, about another 30 minutes.

Pulse chop the coriander. Stir in ½ of the coriander and all the salt. Cook another 1 to 2 minutes. Spoon Tagine over couscous, and garnish with remaining coriander.

YIELD: 4 SERVINGS

1 cup lentils, sorted and washed (see page 199)

3 cups vegetable stock or purified water

2 cloves garlic, peeled

1 carrot, trimmed and quartered

1 yam, scrubbed and quartered

8 pearl onions or 1 yellow onion, peeled and quartered

¼ cup lemon juice, fresh preferred

½ teaspoon ground ginger

½ teaspoon ground coriander

½ teaspoon ground cinnamon

½ teaspoon ground pepper

1 bunch fresh coriander, thick stems removed

1 teaspoon sea salt

1 recipe Savory Saffron Couscous (page 60)

Enchiladas Squared

This recipe is a deep-dish version of your favorite enchiladas—full of south of the border flavor. The pinto beans and corn tortillas provide a complete protein, giving you a meal in one dish—a great casserole to have on hand for lunch. Add a green salad for some crunch!

Soak ½ cup sorted and washed beans in purified water (see page 195).

1 cup soaked beans, like pinto or kidney (½ cup dry) (see Note)

2 cups purified water

1 bay leaf

2 fresh tomatoes, quartered

1 onion, peeled and quartered

1 clove garlic, peeled

1 red bell pepper, seeded and quartered

1 green bell pepper, seeded and quartered

1 tablespoon chili powder

1 teaspoon ground cumin

½ teaspoon sea salt

½ cup ricotta cheese, organic preferred

½ cup plain yogurt with active cultures

¾ cup Monterey Jack cheese, organic preferred

1 teaspoon extra virgin olive oil

12 corn tortillas

Drain the beans from the soaking water. Place into a large saucepan. Add 2 cups purified water and bay leaf. Bring to a boil, covered, and cook for 35 minutes.

Using a blender or food processor, pulse chop the tomatoes, onion, garlic, and peppers. Add the vegetables to the beans, along with the chili powder, cumin, and salt. Return to a boil, lower flame, and simmer, covered, another 10 minutes.

In a medium bowl, blender or food processor, combine ricotta and yogurt. Pulse chop or grate the Monterey Jack.

PREHEAT OVEN TO 350 DEGREES.

Grease a deep 9- x 13-inch baking pan with the oil. Layer 3 or 4 tortillas on the bottom, followed by ⅓ of the bean mixture, ½ cup ricotta-yogurt mixture, and ⅓ of the Jack cheese. Repeat layering process. End with the remainder of the sauce and grated cheese.

Place in the oven, uncovered, and bake for 15 to 20 minutes. Remove from oven, and allow to set 5 minutes before serving.

Cut into large squares and serve.

YIELD: 4 SERVINGS

HEALTHFUL HINT: Don't skip meals. This habit will slow your metabolic rate and cause you to gain weight more easily, causing osteoarthritis of the weight-bearing joints.

NOTE: Any cooked beans left over from another day can be used to make this dish and will reduce preparation time.

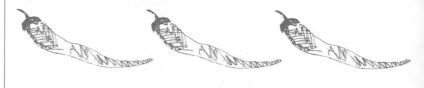

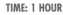
Texas-Inspired Chili

If your family thinks they don't like vegetarian dishes, let them think again. This full flavored chili is not only healthy, but has a hearty taste that'll keep them asking for more.

Drain beans and place in a large saucepan. Add 3 cups water and bay leaf, and bring to a boil, covered. Lower flame and simmer until tender, about 30 minutes.

In a blender or food processor, pulse chop the onion and garlic. Add to the beans along with the chili, cumin, oregano, and cayenne. Increase the flame, returning the chili to a boil, uncovered.

Pulse chop the tomatoes and red pepper, and stir into beans. Add the bulghur, salt, and pepper. Lower heat, cover, and simmer until chili is thick and fragrant, about 20 minutes. Stir occasionally, and add more water, if needed. Pulse chop the red onion and cilantro. Place in a small bowl.

Stir butter into chili, allowing it to melt. Taste and adjust seasoning. Serve in a large individual bowl with cilantro-onion mixture and yogurt on the side, and a bottle of hot sauce, for those who indulge!

YIELD: 4 TEXAN SERVINGS

HEALTHFUL HINT: Red peppers and tomatoes are sources of carotenoids and vitamin C, which provide antioxidants, the antidotes to unstable singlet oxygen molecules, called free-radicals.

NOTE: If you have chipotle chiles left over from the Latin Split Pea Soup recipe, use them here, too. Just soak one in water for 15 minutes, remove the stem and seeds, and pulse chop it along with the onion and garlic. It will add a rich, almost smoky taste to the chili—one of our favorite flavors.

"Chili's a lot like sex: When it's good, it's great, and even when it's bad, it's not so bad."

—Bill Boldenweck

Soak ½ cup sorted and washed beans in purified water (see page 195).

1 cup soaked beans, like pinto or kidney (½ cup dry)

3 cups purified water

1 bay leaf

1 onion, peeled and quartered

3 cloves garlic, peeled

1 tablespoon chili powder (see Note)

1 teaspoon cumin

1 teaspoon oregano

⅛ teaspoon cayenne pepper (optional)

2 ripe tomatoes, quartered

1 sweet red pepper, seeded and quartered

½ cup bulghur wheat

1 teaspoon sea salt

½ teaspoon ground pepper

1 small red onion, peeled and quartered

½ bunch cilantro, thick stems removed

2 tablespoons unsalted butter or extra virgin olive oil

1 cup plain yogurt with active cultures, organic preferred

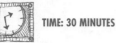

Indian-Style Curried Eggs

Memorable seasonings can make the difference to a restricted diet. These curried eggs are unlike anything you've experienced before—and new studies actually say that eggs are good for you! Accompany this recipe with rice pilaf or couscous, and serve as an entree.

1 almond-sized knob fresh ginger root

6 button mushrooms

6 scallions, trimmed and quartered

2 tablespoons unsalted butter

⅛ teaspoon cayenne pepper

1 ripe tomato, quartered

¼ teaspoon ground turmeric

½ teaspoon ground cumin

8 eggs, organic preferred

¼ cup plain yogurt or buttermilk with active cultures

½ teaspoon sea salt

⅛ teaspoon ground pepper

Fresh coriander or parsley sprigs for garnish

In a blender or food processor, finely pulse chop the ginger. Add the mushrooms and scallions, chopping finely. Melt the butter in a large skillet, over medium heat. Add the ginger mixture and cayenne. Sauté, tossing often, until mushrooms are tender, about 10 minutes.

Pulse chop the tomato. Add to the skillet with the turmeric and cumin. Cook on medium heat, covered, until the tomato is tender, about 3 more minutes.

In a large bowl or blender, whisk the eggs with yogurt or buttermilk, salt, and pepper.

Pour the egg mixture into the skillet with the vegetables. Cook uncovered, stirring constantly with a large spoon, until the eggs are set, yet very creamy. Don't let them dry out. Serve immediately, garnish with coriander or parsley sprigs.

YIELD: 4 SERVINGS

French Red Lentil Pâté

Pâté is usually served as an appetizer, but served with a grain, can make a lovely dinner presentation. The next day slide a slice of cold pâté on top of whole grain bread with a smear of mustard for a terrific lunch.

PREHEAT THE OVEN TO 375 DEGREES

Place the lentils and water or stock in a large saucepan. Bring to a boil on a high flame, covered. Meanwhile, in a blender or food processor, pulse mince the onion and garlic. Add to the lentils. Reduce flame and simmer, stirring occasionally, until the lentils are soft and the water is absorbed, about 30 minutes.

Oil a loaf pan and sprinkle with just enough bread crumbs to coat. Set aside.

Coarsley pulse chop the parsley and ¼ cup sunflower seeds. Add to the beans along with the herbal salt, pepper, oil or butter, and ½ cup bread crumbs. Mix well. The pâté should be very thick. If needed, add any remaining bread crumbs.

Pour the pâté into the loaf pan and smooth the top. Sprinkle the remaining sunflower seeds on top of the loaf and press gently into the beans. Place the loaf in the oven and bake until browned and the edges are slightly pulled away from the sides, about 30 minutes.

Remove the loaf from the oven, and allow to cool about 10 minutes. Turn the loaf onto a cutting board or serving platter. Cut into slices and serve while warm.

HEALTHFUL HINT: Some people shy away from using seeds and nuts in recipes because of their perceived high calorie/high fat contents. Yet seeds and nuts are an excellent source of nourishment, so do use them. They're packed with vitamins and minerals, as well as essential fats that are good for your joints.

2 cups red lentils, sorted and washed

4 cups purified water or any unsalted stock (except fish)

1 onion, peeled and quartered

3 cloves garlic, peeled

3 tablespoons extra virgin olive oil or unsalted butter

¾ cup whole grain bread crumbs

½ bunch fresh parsley, thick stems removed and washed

½ cup raw sunflower seeds

2 teaspoons herbal sea salt

½ teaspoon ground white pepper

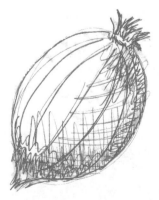

Chicken and Turkey

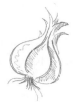

Stuffed Chicken Breasts Florentine Style

Braised Chicken with Hazelnuts, Prunes, and Apricots

Creamy Tarragon Chicken

Garlicky Oven-Fried Chicken

Singapore-Style Chicken with Satay Sauce

Roasted Chicken Smothered with Prosciutto

Citrusy Herb Chicken with Creamy Yogurt Sauce

The Tangiest Teriyaki Chicken

Chicken 'n Healthy Dumplings with Horseradish Sauce

Roasted Breast of Turkey with Tarragon and Lemon

Gourmet Turkey-Apple Loaf

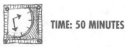 **TIME: 50 MINUTES**

Stuffed Chicken Breasts Florentine Style

A rich tasting recipe doesn't have to be loaded with fat. In this dish, fragrant herbs and spices are used to infuse spinach-stuffed chicken breasts for a decidedly Tuscan taste.

1 bunch fresh spinach, thick stems removed and washed (about 4 packed cups)

½ cup purified water

¼ onion, peeled

2 anchovies or 8 oil-cured black olives, pitted

1 egg, organic preferred

2 tablespoons extra virgin olive oil

1 teaspoon dried thyme

⅛ teaspoon ground nutmeg

½ teaspoon herbal sea salt

⅛ teaspoon ground pepper

4 chicken breast cutlets, organic preferred (see Note)

2 tablespoons lemon juice

1 teaspoon dried rosemary

½ cup chicken stock, homemade preferred, or purified water

NOTE: The cutlets need a pocket cut into each one—ask your butcher to do this step. If you weren't able to have the pockets cut for you, the cutlets can be arranged in the pan with the spinach filling placed on top. Then change the name to Un-Stuffed Chicken Breasts!

PREHEAT OVEN TO 450 DEGREES.

Place spinach and water in a 2-quart saucepan. Cover, bring to a boil, and reduce flame. Simmer until the spinach is wilted, about 3 minutes. Drain, and set aside to cool.

In a blender or food processor, pulse chop the ¼ onion, and anchovies or olives. Place in a medium bowl.

Press or squeeze out all the excess spinach liquid, and pulse chop. Add the egg, blending well. Add to the onion mixture along with the oil, thyme, nutmeg, ¼ teaspoon herbal salt, and pepper. Mix well.

Using a paring knife, slit the chicken breast on the thickest side, making a pocket. Stuff spinach filling into pocket. Do not overfill. Place breasts in a baking dish. Close with a wooden toothpick, if desired.

Pour stock over breasts. Sprinkle chicken with lemon juice, rosemary, and ¼ teaspoon salt.

Cover with parchment paper and then foil. Place in oven and cook for 30 minutes. Uncover and continue cooking until lightly browned, and the juices run clear when pierced with a fork, about 10 to 15 minutes more. Serve with rice pilaf.

YIELD: 4 SERVINGS

HEALTHFUL HINT: Animal products such as chicken are high in phosphorous. Arthritis patients taking NSAID medications, which trigger the body to excrete phosphorous, may need to replenish their supply with phosphorous-high foods.

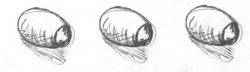

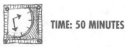

THE ARTHRITIS CURE COOKBOOK

Braised Chicken with Hazelnuts, Prunes, and Apricots

Sweet and savory flavors together can be very satisfying. Getting an appropriate amount of nutrients for your body can be easy with tasty, well balanced recipes such as this.

Wash the chicken in cold water and dry thoroughly with paper toweling. Heat the oil in a large skillet on a medium-high flame. Add the chicken pieces and dust with salt and pepper. Cook each side until golden brown, using tongs to turn the pieces over, about 5 to 7 minutes per side. After turning, season the uncooked side with additional salt and pepper. Transfer the golden brown chicken to a plate and cover.

In a small skillet over medium flame, lightly toast hazelnuts for 2 to 3 minutes, stirring frequently. Be careful not to burn. Remove to a bowl and let cool.

In a small processor pulse chop the hazelnuts into coarse pieces. Return all but 1 tablespoon of the nut pieces back to the bowl. Grind remaining tablespoon into a fine meal or powder. Set aside. In a blender or food processor, pulse mince the garlic and onions.

Drain off all but 3 tablespoons of the oil from cooking the chicken. Add the garlic and onion to the skillet and sauté until softened and golden, about 10 minutes. Add ½ cup stock, the prunes, apricots, oregano, and cumin. Reduce heat and simmer, covered, for 4 or 5 minutes.

Add the chopped and finely ground hazelnuts, capers, and the remaining stock. Stir. Bring the liquid to a boil. Reduce heat, cover. Simmer for 5 minutes.

Return the chicken to the skillet. Coat the chicken evenly with sauce, cover, and cook thoroughly, about 5 more minutes.

Arrange the chicken on a serving platter. Taste the sauce and adjust seasoning, if needed. Pour sauce over chicken. Serve with buttered udon noodles and a salad.

YIELD: 4 SERVINGS

3 tablespoons extra virgin olive oil

One 3½-pound fryer chicken, organic preferred, cut into 8 to 10 pieces

Sea salt

Ground pepper

¼ cup raw hazelnuts

3 cloves garlic, peeled

2 onions, peeled and quartered

1 ½ cups chicken stock, homemade preferred, or purified water

½ cup prunes, unsulphured preferred

½ cup apricots, unsulphured preferred

½ teaspoon dried oregano

¼ teaspoon ground cumin

2 tablespoons capers

HEALTHFUL HINT: An important mineral contained in our bones is potassium. Dried fruits such as prunes and apricots are a good source of this needed mineral. Many dried fruits are preserved in sulphur dioxide to retain their color and moisture. Look for the brands without this harmful chemical. (Hint: the fruits will be a darker color.)

TIME: 55 MINUTES

Creamy Tarragon Chicken

This creamy dish, made with yogurt, is satisfying and yet slimming. Maintaining proper body weight has a bonus for arthritis sufferers. Less weight on the body means fewer pounds resting on hip and knee joints.

2 teaspoons unsalted butter

One 2½- to 3-pound chicken, quartered

3 cloves garlic, peeled

2 sprigs fresh or 1½ teaspoons dried tarragon

1¼ cups chicken stock, homemade preferred or purified water

½ teaspoon sea salt

¼ teaspoon ground pepper

¾ cup plain yogurt with active cultures

1½ tablespoons whole wheat flour

3 sprigs parsley, leaves only, washed and pulse chopped

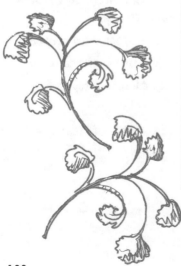

PREHEAT OVEN TO 375 DEGREES.

Grease a deep 9- x 13-inch baking pan with ½ teaspoon butter. Place the chicken in the pan, bone side down. Bake until the chicken has browned, about 30 minutes. It will not be thoroughly cooked.

In a blender or food processor, pulse mince the garlic and tarragon. Heat a medium-size skillet on a medium-high flame, with the remaining 1½ teaspoons butter, and sauté the garlic and tarragon briefly. Add the stock, salt, and pepper. On a high flame, bring liquid to a boil, covered. Reduce the heat and simmer 5 minutes.

Using tongs, remove the chicken from the oven to the skillet. Spoon the sauce over the chicken, cover, and cook until the juices run clear when inserted with a fork, about 20 minutes. Baste occasionally.

In a small bowl, combine yogurt and flour.

Remove the chicken to a serving platter and cover, or place in the oven to keep warm.

Add 2 tablespoons of the tarragon sauce to yogurt mixture and stir well. Add several more tablespoons of sauce, stirring again. Using a whisk, add the yogurt mixture to skillet, blending well. Cook until the sauce bubbles and is hot, whisking constantly, about 1 or 2 more minutes.

Pour the sauce over the chicken and sprinkle with parsley. Serve with baked yams.

YIELD: 4 SERVINGS

HEALTHFUL HINT: Providing good quality fats, such as extra virgin olive oil, unsalted butter, and flax seed oil, in small amounts in your meals daily, will actually reduce your total food consumption by allowing you to feel satisfied and full faster—thus eating less quantity

Garlicky Oven-Fried Chicken

This entree has all the taste of its fried cousin, but is a much healthier alternative that uses garlic to give it a truly decadent taste. For those who like to entertain, this dish has all the makings of a crowd pleaser—and leftovers will be a real pleasure!

PREHEAT OVEN TO 400 DEGREES.

In a blender or food blender, pulse mince the garlic. In a medium bowl, combine the garlic with the bread crumbs, cornmeal, sesame seeds, ½ teaspoon salt, and ¼ teaspoon pepper. Mix well.

In a small bowl, mix the mustard, water, and molasses together. Add an extra pinch each of the salt and pepper.

Coat each piece of chicken with the mustard mixture, then dip the pieces in the bread crumbs and coat evenly.

Place the chicken on a lightly greased baking sheet, bone side down. Bake until crisp and browned, and the juices run clear when inserted with a fork, about 40 to 45 minutes.

Serve hot, at room temperature, or chilled with picnic salad goodies.

YIELD: 4 SERVINGS

HEALTHFUL HINT: Chicken and other foods that are prepared deep-fried come with an extra dose of free-radicals, generated by heating certain oils to the high temperatures of frying. Free-radicals are those mini-molecules that attack and break down our bodies on the cellular level, including the subtle structures of bone joints. Don't fry in fat—bake instead!

> *"Eat plenty of garlic. This guarantees you twelve hours of sleep—alone—every night."*
>
> —Chris Chase

5 cloves garlic, peeled

1⅓ cups whole grain bread crumbs (see Note)

2 tablespoons high-lysine cornmeal

2 tablespoons unhulled sesame seeds

½ teaspoon sea salt, plus extra

¼ teaspoon ground pepper, plus extra

2 tablespoons Dijon-style mustard

1 tablespoon purified water

2 teaspoons unsulphured blackstrap molasses, real maple syrup, or honey

One 2½- to 3-pound chicken, organic preferred, cut into 8 pieces

NOTE: To make your own bread crumbs, toast 3 slices whole grain bread, cut or break into pieces, and pulverize in a blender or food processor. Whole grain bread crumbs are available in the natural food store, and these are minus the sugar, the hydrogenated fats, and the preservatives.

Singapore-Style Chicken with Satay Sauce

This is the healthy version of the entree found in many Thai and Indonesian restaurants. In this simple preparation, this dish is downright beneficial and also easy to prepare.

Prepare the marinade, and marinate the chicken for 2 hours.

2 garlic cloves, peeled

¼ cup imported soy sauce

3 tablespoons sesame or extra virgin olive oil

2 teaspoons curry powder

2 teaspoons honey or real maple syrup

4 chicken cutlets, organic preferred

1 recipe Satay Sauce (see page 164)

"My tongue is smiling."
—Abigail Trillin

TO PREPARE THE MARINADE:

In a blender or food processor, pulse mince the garlic. Put the garlic in a medium bowl with the soy sauce, oil, curry powder, and honey. Stir well.

Cut the chicken into ¾-inch cubes. Add to the soy marinade, tossing the pieces to coat evenly.

Cover the bowl with plastic film and place in the refrigerator. Marinate for at least 2 hours or overnight, turning the chicken occasionally.

TO COOK THE CHICKEN:

Using bamboo skewers, thread the chicken cubes onto the skewers, leaving 1 to 1½ inches at the blunt end of each skewer, to facilitate handling.

PREHEAT THE BROILER.

Position the oven rack about 3 inches from the broiler heat source.

Cook the chicken about 2 inches from the heat, or cook on a grill if desired. Turn frequently, cooking until the chicken is golden brown, about 8 minutes.

Arrange the skewers on a serving platter. Serve with Satay Sauce on the side.

YIELD: 4 SERVINGS

Roasted Chicken Smothered with Prosciutto

While savory meats such as prosciutto may not find their way into your every-day diet, it is a perfect occasional treat to a healthful menu. In this savory tasting dish, low-fat vegetables and herbs are baked with the chicken, taking advantage of the meat's natural flavors.

PREHEAT OVEN TO 350 DEGREES.

In a blender or food processor, pulse chop the celery, garlic, onion, carrot, and parsley.

In medium-size skillet, heat the oil on a moderate flame and add the vegetables and sage. Pulse chop prosciutto and add. Sauté until the onions begin to clear, about 5 to 7 minutes.

Place the vegetable mixture on the bottom of a deep 9- x 13-inch baking dish. Add the stock. Put the chicken top of the vegetables, bone side down. Season chicken with a dusting of salt and pepper.

Bake chicken until tender when inserted with a fork and the juices run clear, about 40 to 45 minutes. Turn chicken over in the last 10 minutes of cooking. Serve with a salad and baked yams.

Smother with prosciutto sauce.

YIELD: 4 SERVINGS

HEALTHFUL HINT: Roasting a chicken requires little effort and can provide delicious leftovers for labor-saving meals.

3 celery ribs, quartered

3 garlic cloves, peeled

1 onion, peeled and quartered

1 carrot, trimmed and quartered

4 sprigs fresh parsley, thick stems removed

2 tablespoons extra virgin olive oil

½ teaspoon sage

4 slices Italian prosciutto ham

1½ cups hot chicken stock, homemade preferred, or purified water

One 3- to 3½-pound chicken, organic preferred, quartered

Sea salt

Ground pepper

"No one can love his neighbor on an empty stomach."

—Woodrow Wilson

Citrusy Herbed Chicken with Creamy Yogurt Sauce

Marinate chicken to create a creative and tasty dinner with its distinctly Middle-Eastern essence. This recipe is not only delicious, but also extremely healthy.

Prepare the marinade, and marinate the chicken for 4 hours or overnight.

1 lemon, organic preferred

½ cup lemon juice, fresh preferred

4 tablespoons extra virgin olive oil

½ cup unsweetened apple juice

½ teaspoon sea salt

¼ teaspoon ground pepper

2 sprigs fresh rosemary, thick stems removed, or 1 teaspoon dried

2 sprigs fresh thyme, thick stems removed, or 1 teaspoon dried

½ bunch fresh parsley, thick stems removed

4 chicken cutlets, organic preferred

2 tablespoons unsalted butter

½ cup plain yogurt with active cultures, organic preferred

1 bunch watercress

HEALTHFUL HINT: Lemons have the most bioflavonoids of any citrus, so it's a good idea to use them in various dishes, since bioflavonoids have been found to strengthen joints. And for those who want the most benefit from the bioflavonoids, eat a wedge of the cooked lemon, the skin, pith, and flesh—if you dare!!

TO PREPARE THE MARINADE: Cut the lemon into 8 pieces and place in a non metallic container with a lid. Add lemon juice, 2 tablespoons oil, apple juice, salt, and pepper. In a small processor mince the rosemary and thyme. Add to the marinade. Pulse chop the parsley and add half to the marinade. Set remainder aside. Stir marinade to blend.

Place the chicken in the marinade, and spoon some of the liquid on top. Cover and place in the refrigerator. Marinate at least 4 hours.

TO COOK THE CHICKEN: Remove the chicken pieces from marinade to a plate. Using paper toweling, pat them dry on all sides. Set aside.

In a large sauté pan over medium-high heat, melt the butter and remaining 2 tablespoons oil. Add the chicken and sauté until golden brown on both sides, turning once. The chicken should be tender when inserted with a fork and the juices will run clear, at least 7 minutes per side. Transfer cutlets to a clean dish and cover to keep warm.

Discard excess butter and oil from the pan. Add marinade to the pan, and bring to a boil. Cook uncovered, reducing to about ½ cup. Add several tablespoons of the hot marinade to the yogurt and stir well. Pour yogurt into pan and simmer just until warm, about 1 minute. Do not boil. Taste, and add salt and pepper, if needed. Add remaining parsley and stir.

Return chicken to the pan and spoon sauce over top. Cover and heat thoroughly, about 1 minute.

Place chicken on platter, and garnish with watercress.

YIELD: 4 SERVINGS

The Tangiest Teriyaki Chicken

Marinades are a labor-saving way to add flavor to everyday dishes. In this recipe, we borrow the flavors of the Far East to provide an update to easy-to-prepare baked chicken.

TO PREPARE THE MARINADE: In a blender or food processor, pulse mince the garlic and ginger. Put in a small bowl with the soy sauce, oil, water, molasses, mustard, and vinegar. Mix well.

In a deep 9- x 13-inch baking pan place the chicken and pour the marinade over. Cover with plastic film and refrigerate. Marinate for at least 1 hour, turning twice.

TO COOK THE CHICKEN: Place the chicken and ½ cup marinade in a large sauté pan. Bring to a boil, covered, lower flame, and cook until the chicken is tender when inserted with a fork and the juices run clear, about 30 minutes.

Preheat the broiler.

Put chicken on a baking sheet, skin side up. Broil until golden brown, about 4 to 5 minutes. Serve immediately.

YIELD: 4 SERVINGS

Prepare the marinade, and marinate the chicken for at least 1 hour.

3 garlic cloves, peeled

1 walnut-sized knob fresh ginger root

½ cup imported soy sauce

¼ cup sesame or extra virgin olive oil

¼ cup purified water or unsweetened apple juice

3 tablespoons unsulphured blackstrap molasses

2 tablespoons Dijon mustard

2 tablespoons cider vinegar

One 3- to 3½-pound chicken, cut in 8 pieces

HEALTHFUL HINT: Ginger is beneficial to the digestion by aiding in the breakdown of fatty foods, preventing flatulence, and stimulating the liver. Thus it is especially useful when eaten with chicken, beans, or other meats. Good digestion is important in order to absorb all the important arthritis-friendly nutrients.

STASH & SNACK

Chicken 'n Healthy Dumplings with Horseradish Sauce

Not at all the dish your mom used to make! This really healthy and delicious version of an old classic has all the nutrients and flavor—and very little fat.

One 3- to 4-pound chicken, quartered

2 quarts purified water

1 teaspoon cider vinegar

2 onions, peeled and quartered

1 carrot, trimmed and quartered

2 teaspoons sea salt

1 teaspoon ground pepper

½ bunch parsley, thick stems removed and washed

2 cloves garlic, peeled

3 eggs, organic preferred

1 cup buttermilk (see Note 1)

1 teaspoon herbal sea salt

1 teaspoon baking soda

About 2 to 2½ cups whole wheat pastry flour

½ cup plain yogurt with active cultures

1 to 2 teaspoons prepared horseradish

NOTE 1: The buttermilk can be substituted with ¾ cup yogurt and ¼ cup purified water.

Place the chicken pieces in a Dutch oven and add the water, vinegar, 1 onion, carrot, 2 teaspoons salt, and ¼ teaspoon pepper. Add half the parsley sprigs. Pulse chop the remaining parsley, onion, and garlic. Remove to a bowl, and set aside. Cover the pot and bring to a boil. Lower flame and simmer until chicken is tender and the juices run clear when pierced with a fork, about 40 minutes.

Prepare the dumpling batter about 10 minutes before chicken is finished cooking.

In a blender or processor, blend the eggs, buttermilk, herbal salt, soda, and ¼ teaspoon pepper. Blend until smooth. Add 1 cup flour, and blend mixture again. Add ½ cup more flour and blend. Add remaining flour, ¼ cup at a time, blending after each addition.

Pour the batter into the bowl with the reserved onion mixture, and mix well. Add additional flour until the dough is stiff enough to be pushed off the spoon with a rubber spatula.

HEALTHFUL HINT: Poaching a chicken releases the gelatinous substance in its bones. Th gelatin has been found to strengthen arthritic joints. The added vinegar draws calcium fro the bones into the broth.

Using a slotted spoon, carefully remove chicken to a heat-proof serving container with a lid. Cover and keep in a warm area.

Return the pot to a boil, on a high flame. Using 2 teaspoons, drop spoonsful of dumpling dough. Circle the outside of the pot, and then continue to drop balls in the center. At first they will sink, and as they begin to cook, the dumplings will float to the surface. Cook in 2 batches.

Cook covered, on a medium-high flame, for 15 minutes. (A cooked dumpling will be solidified, doughy, and chewy on the inside, not runney or gooey.) (see Note 2).

In a small bowl, mix together the yogurt and horseradish.

Serve the chicken on a platter with the dumplings. Put the horseradish sauce in a bowl on the side.

YIELD: 4 SERVINGS

NOTE 2: The stock that gets created from cooking this chicken and dumpling recipe is perfectly good to use as a base for a soup. We added a few squeezes of lemon and served it as a broth the next day. It has become a family favorite!

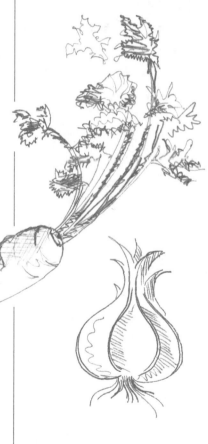

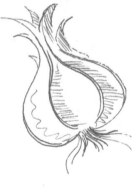

"A Chicken in Every Pot."
—Herbert Hoover campaign slogan

Roasted Breast of Turkey with Tarragon and Lemon

Turkey can now be eaten year-round. Enjoy this Thanksgiving favorite, whenever the mood strikes you.

1 turkey breast or half (see Note)

1 lemon, cut in half

Sea salt

Ground pepper

Tarragon leaves

NOTE: The butcher can cut a fresh or frozen turkey in half, and the second half can be stored in the freezer for later use.

PREHEAT OVEN TO 425 DEGREES.

Place the turkey breast or half in a roasting pan, bone side up. Squeeze ½ lemon all over. Lightly sprinkle with salt, pepper, and tarragon. Turn turkey over, skin side up and repeat with the lemon and spices.

Place in the oven and reduce heat to 350 degrees. Roast uncovered, allowing 20 minutes per pound. The juice should run clear when a thick area (such as the breast or thigh) is pierced with a fork. The skin will be brown.

YIELD: 4 SERVINGS

HEALTHFUL HINT: Vitamin A is an antioxidant which is important in an anti-osteoarthrit diet to quench free radicals. Turkey is high in vitamin A.

TIME: 1 HOUR, 5 MINUTES

Gourmet Turkey-Apple Loaf

An updated version of an old favorite, this meat loaf is a healthy and hearty entree. Leftover slices make great sandwiches.

PREHEAT OVEN TO 350 DEGREES.

In a blender or food processor, pulse mince the apples, onion, garlic, and parsley.

Melt the butter in a medium skillet, on a moderate flame. Add the apple mixture. Cook until the onions are translucent, about 5 minutes. Stir frequently. Remove from the flame and cool.

In a large bowl or processor, mix the apple mixture, turkey, oats, eggs, mustard, marjoram, sage, salt, and pepper.

Lightly oil a 9- x 5-inch loaf pan. Pat the turkey mixture into the pan. Bake until the top is golden, about 1 hour.

Remove the loaf from the oven, pour off any excess fat, and invert onto a platter. Slice and serve.

YIELD: 4 SERVINGS

HEALTHFUL HINT: Ground turkey from the supermarket often contains turkey skin, which increases its fat content substantially. For the leanest ground turkey, call ahead and ask the butcher to grind skinless turkey breast for you. It will be ready to pick up when you get there.

"Things don't change. You just change your way of looking, that's all."

—Carlos Castaneda

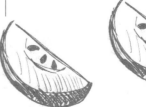

2 Granny Smith or Macintosh apples, quartered and core removed

1 onion, peeled and quartered

1 garlic clove, peeled

½ bunch fresh parsley, thick stems removed and washed (see Note)

2 teaspoons unsalted butter

1½ pounds lean ground turkey

½ cup rolled oats or whole grain bread crumbs

2 eggs, organic preferred

1 teaspoon Dijon mustard

¾ teaspoon marjoram

½ teaspoon sage

1 teaspoon sea salt

½ teaspoon ground pepper

NOTE: Treat yourself to an electric mini-chopper for cutting small amounts of greens such as the parsley in this recipe.

Fish and Shellfish

Grilled Swordfish with Mango-Papaya Salsa

Long Island Soft-Shell Crabs

Asian-Style Sesame Sea Bass

Shrimp a la Greque

Updated Scallop and Shrimp Seviche

Catfish Stew with Cornmeal Wedges

Fettuccini Italiana alla Salmone

Emerald Zuppa de Pesci

Caldo de Ostiones

Mediterranean Fillet of Sole Almondine

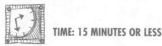
Grilled Swordfish with Mango-Papaya Salsa

Tasty and easy-to-fix, this recipe combines the delicate flavor of swordfish with tropical tastes. Fresh swordfish is available for much of the year. It has a better flavor than packaged frozen fish and more of its healthful benefits for you to absorb. It's a wonderfully light dish to prepare for summer entertaining and a genuine treat for any meal. (Try it with or without the Papaya-Mango Salsa—a hit either way!)

Prepare salsa, up to 2 days in advance.

4 half-inch-thick swordfish steaks

1 tablespoon unsalted butter

Sea salt

Ground pepper

1 recipe Papaya-Mango Salsa, room temperature (page 161)

NOTE: The fish steaks can also be grilled, for a wonderful flavor.

Position the oven rack about 4 inches from the broiler heat source. Preheat the broiler (see Note).

Place fish steaks in a greased, nonglass baking pan. Dot fish with remaining butter, and dust with salt and pepper.

Broil the fish until it begins to flake and has no resistance when a fork is inserted, about 3 or 4 minutes. Be watchful that it doesn't burn. Do not turn the fish over.

Using a spatula, place fish steaks on individual plates and spoon several tablespoons of the Papaya-Mango Salsa on top. Serve hot or cold.

YIELD: 4 SERVINGS

HEALTHFUL HINT: Richly flavored fish such as swordfish, salmon, and tuna are full of nutritious fish oils that reduce inflammation by reducing inflammatory leukotrienes.

"To live is so startling it leaves little time for anything else."
—Emily Dickinson

Long Island Soft-Shell Crabs

Many people remember a time when seafood was only for special occasions. Due to new methods of farming and cultivating shellfish, wider varieties of seafood are now readily available and reasonably priced. Soft-shell crabs are in season May through September. They are easy to cook, and can make an ordinary meal seem like a *very* special occasion.

In a shallow, wide bowl mix the flour, salt, pepper, and sage. Wash the cleaned crabs in cold water and individually toss them in the flour mixture, coating lightly. Place each on a plate, and continue coating the crabs until all are done.

In a large sauté pan (large enough to fit all the crabs at once), heat half the butter and oil. Add the crabs, cover with a splatter guard, and cook over medium heat until crabs start to turn pink, about 5 to 7 minutes. (Be careful not to get burned, as they tend to spit and pop.)

Meanwhile, juice 2 lemons and cut 1 into wedges. Set aside.

Add remaining butter and oil. Using tongs, carefully turn crabs and cook on the other side, another 4 to 5 minutes.

Have the cover of the pan nearby. Pour juice over crabs and immediately cover. Steam for 1 or 2 minutes. Serve immediately with lemon wedges on the side.

YIELD: 4 SERVINGS

HEALTHFUL HINT: These are an excellent source of calcium, because soft-shell crabs, calcium-rich shells and all, can be eaten in their entirety. A calcium deficiency may induce aching joints, rheumatoid arthritis, and insomnia.

1 cup whole wheat flour
or high-lysine cornmeal

¼ teaspoon sea salt

½ teaspoon ground pepper

Pinch sage

4 soft-shell crabs (see Note)

3 tablespoons unsalted
butter

3 tablespoons extra-virgin
olive oil

3 lemons

NOTE: Buy and use fish and shellfish the same day. For the freshest crabs, make sure they are alive before purchasing, and have your fish monger clean them for you.

"Cooking is like love. It should be entered into with abandon or not at all."
—Harriet Van Horne

Asian-Style Sesame Sea Bass

The exotic flavors of this delightful dish come from the unique marriage of some very common Asian ingredients. The sesame oil imparts the distinctive rich, nutty flavor of this dish, while cilantro, fresh ginger, soy sauce, and scallions give the fish a wonderful savory and spicy flavor.

One 3- to 4-pound whole sea bass, cleaned

1 walnut-sized knob fresh ginger root

3 tablespoons imported soy sauce

3 scallions, trimmed and quartered

2 stems cilantro, thick stems removed and washed

2 tablespoons dark sesame oil

HEALTHFUL HINT: Dark sesame oil is made from roasted sesame seeds. It is healthiest when added after the fish is out of the oven to avoid exposing it to the high baking temperatures, which can break down oils into unhealthy free-radicals that can wear away at joints and connective tissue.

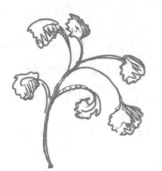

PREHEAT OVEN TO 425 DEGREES.

Lay out one large piece of parchment paper or heavy-duty aluminum foil. Wash the fish in cold water, removing any scales and loose tissues from the cavity. Place fish on top of the paper or foil.

In a blender or food processor, pulse mince the ginger. Drizzle the soy sauce over fish and in the cavity, and scatter with ginger.

Note thickness of the fish to determine approximate cooking time. Fold the paper or foil together to form a tightly closed packet, with an interior air space between the top of the fish and the closure. Seal tightly. If necessary, place the parchment package in a large sheet of foil to further ensure the closure. Place the package on a baking sheet.

Bake the fish until cooked thoroughly, allowing 10 to 12 minutes of cooking time for each inch of fish thickness. Test by carefully opening the package and inserting a fork into the thickest part of the fish. Be cautious to avoid the hot steam that will escape. The fork should slide in easily, having no resistance. Remove the fish from the oven if done, or reclose and cook several more minutes.

Pulse chop the scallions and cilantro.

Using two spatulas, carefully remove the baked fish from the parchment or foil to a serving platter.

Drizzle sea bass with oil and pour cooking juices over the fish. Sprinkle with scallions and cilantro. Serve immediately.

YIELD: 4 SERVINGS

Shrimp a la Greque

This is a remarkably easy-to-prepare version of a shrimp dish you can order in the fancier restaurants. Impress your family or guests with your culinary prowess by taking in an afternoon matinee and whipping up this culinary delight in less time than it takes to set the table!

PREHEAT OVEN TO 425 DEGREES.

In a blender or food processor, pulse chop the garlic, parsley, and onion. In a medium sauté pan, on a high flame, heat the olive oil and butter. Add the vegetables, and cook until lightly browned, about 10 minutes.

Add the shrimp, oregano, salt, and pepper. Sauté until shrimp turns pink.

Add the lemon juice and cook another 30 seconds. Serve immediately with Babe's Real Greek Pilaf (page 63).

YIELD: 4 SERVINGS

4 garlic cloves, peeled

3 sprigs fresh parsley, thick stems removed and washed

1 onion, peeled and quartered

2 tablespoons extra virgin olive oil

2 tablespoons unsalted butter

1 pound shrimp, peeled and deveined

1 tablespoon dried oregano

¼ teaspoon sea salt

Pinch ground pepper

2 tablespoons lemon juice

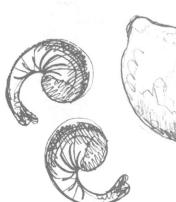

"Man is born to eat."
—Craig Claiborne

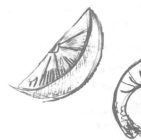

Catfish Stew with Cornmeal Wedges

Catfish is now being farmed in the United States. It is easily available in local markets and can be used to prepare many tasty recipes. Here, it's paired with cornmeal, cooked like cereal, and cut into wedges.

Prepare the Cornmeal Corners up to 5 days ahead of time.

2 onions, peeled and quartered

2 ribs celery, quartered

2 carrots, trimmed and quartered

2 parsnips, trimmed and quartered

1 tablespoon extra virgin olive oil

2 slices bacon, no nitrites preferred

1½ cups fish or chicken stock, homemade preferred, or purified water

½ teaspoon herbal sea salt

¼ teaspoon ground pepper

¼ teaspoon hot pepper sauce (optional)

2 tablespoons lemon juice

1 pound catfish fillets, skinned and boned

1 recipe Midwestern Cornmeal Wedges (see page 57)

In a blender or food processor, pulse chop the onions, celery, carrots, and parsnip. Heat a large Dutch oven on a high flame and add the oil and vegetables. Sauté until soft, about 5 minutes.

In a small frying pan cook the bacon until crisp. Drain on paper toweling.

Add the stock or water, bacon, salt, pepper, and hot pepper sauce to the Dutch oven. Bring to a boil, covered. Lower heat and simmer until the vegetables are cooked, about 10 to 15 minutes.

Add the lemon juice and stir. Place the catfish in pot, and spoon some of the stewed vegetables over it. Continue cooking covered, for another 10 minutes.

Arrange the Midwestern Cornmeal Wedges on individual plates, and spoon stew over. Serve hot.

YIELD: 4 SERVINGS

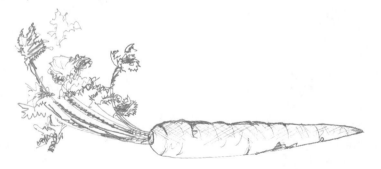

Fettuccini Italiana alla Salmone

It's our opinion that an occasional treat is not only satisfying, it lessens over-indulgence. This recipe is the healthy version of the rich fettuccini dishes that you're always reluctant to order. It has less than half the fat of its restaurant cousin—and our families licked their plates clean. *Buon appetito!*

In a medium frying pan, combine 1 cup water, vinegar, and bay leaf, cover and bring to a boil. Reduce heat to a low flame and add salmon. Cover and poach salmon until opaque and tender when inserted with a fork, about 4 to 6 minutes.

Bring a large pot of water to a boil for the pasta.

Using a slotted spoon or spatula, remove the salmon to a plate and let cool. Discard poaching liquid and bay leaf.

Pulse chop the zucchini, or use the sugar snaps whole. In a small pot, add ½ cup water and zucchini. Bring to a boil, covered, reduce flame and steam until tender, about 3 or 4 minutes. Do not overcook.

In a blender or food processor, combine the cream, yogurt, and nutmeg. Blend until mixed. Pour into a medium frying pan, and heat on a medium-low flame.

Put sea salt into boiling water and add the fettuccini. Cook until just tender or al dente. Drain and transfer to a large serving bowl. Do not rinse.

Cut the salmon into 1-inch chunks. Add to the cream sauce with the zucchini and Romano cheese. Add the pepper and stir, heating until very warm but not boiling.

Pour the cream sauce over the cooked pasta, and toss gently to combine. Serve at once.

YIELD: 4 SERVINGS

1½ cups purified water, plus extra

1 tablespoon cider vinegar

1 bay leaf

1 8-ounce salmon fillet, skin removed

**1 zucchini, quartered, or
1 cup sugar snap peas, tips removed**

½ pint heavy cream, organic preferred

¼ cup plain yogurt with active cultures

¼ teaspoon ground nutmeg

2 teaspoons sea salt

One 8-ounce box whole grain fettuccini or ribbons

1 tablespoon grated Romano cheese

Pinch ground white pepper

HEALTHFUL HINT: Don't fall for spinach or artichoke pastas. They are made with refined semolina flour and are missing the bran and germ—important nutrients that pasta has to offer. The imported whole wheat Italian varieties are very tasty, and there are now several American brands that meet the mark.

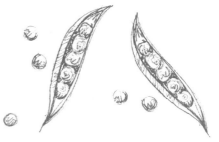

Updated Scallop and Shrimp Seviche

Traditionally, seviche is made with raw fish that has marinated for many hours in lime or lemon juice. The acid of the juices "cook" the fish without heat. These days it's not safe. Use our method of light steaming, and this recipe becomes a welcome light meal or appetizer—and the marinating time gets cut by 4 hours!

½ pound bay scallops

½ pound medium raw shrimp, peeled and deveined

1 cup purified water

Juice of 3 limes, ⅓ to ½ cup

Juice of 3 lemons, ⅓ to ½ cup

2 cloves garlic, peeled

½ red onion, peeled and cut in half

½ bunch parsley, thick stems removed and washed

¼ cup extra-virgin olive oil

½ teaspoon herbal sea salt

¼ teaspoon ground white pepper

1 head Boston lettuce

½ ripe avocado

2 scallions, trimmed and pulse chopped

Rinse scallops and shrimp in cold water and drain. In a medium saucepan, bring the water to a boil. Add the scallops and cover. Cook very briefly, just until the scallops begin to turn opaque, about 2 minutes. Using a slotted spoon, remove them to a bowl and cover with cold water to stop cooking. Repeat the procedure with the shrimp, cooking just until they start to turn pink, about 2 minutes. Remove to the cold water. Pour shellfish into a colander and drain.

Place lime and lemon juices in a medium nonmetallic bowl or container with a lid. Add cooled and drained shellfish, and toss. Make sure that the fish is covered with juice.

In a blender or food processor, pulse mince the garlic, red onion, and parsley. Add to the shellfish along with the oil, herbal salt, and pepper. Cover bowl and refrigerate for at least 1 hour. Stir after 30 minutes.

Carefully separate lettuce leaves. Wash and pat dry with a clean cotton towel; and refrigerate in a plastic bag to keep cool and crisp until ready to use.

HEALTHFUL HINT: Avocados contain beneficial fat that lowers the LDL cholesterol (the lousy one) and increases the HDL (the healthy one). The fat in avocados is the monounsaturated kind, which is high in beneficial anti-inflammatory fatty acids. Here's a food that has fat that is so beneficial, it can be eaten often.

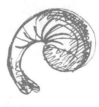

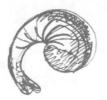

Cut the avocado in half. Using a paring knife, score the side without the seed, in a crosshatched pattern, ½-inch wide. Slide a spoon between the shell and the avocado flesh, and scoop the pieces out. Add them to the shellfish mixture. Stir well. Taste and add salt, if desired (see Note).

Place several lettuce leaves on each individual plate, and scoop seviche into the center. Serve with slices of hearty whole grain bread on the side.

YIELD: 4 SERVINGS

NOTE: The avocado pit helps to keep the unused portion of the flesh from turning brown.

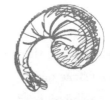

> *"I think that wherever your journey takes you, there are new gods waiting there, with divine patience—and laughter."*
>
> —Susan M. Watkins

Emerald Zuppa de Pesci

This hearty, soupy-stew is loaded with good-for-you fresh herbs and several types of mouth-watering shellfish. A perfect meal served in big, deep bowls with slices of Bruschetta Italiana. A delicious main course, with everything contained in one dish!

12 mussels (see Note)

8 cherrystone clams

½ cup high-lysine cornmeal

1 onion, peeled and quartered

2 garlic cloves, peeled

3 tablespoons extra-virgin olive oil

½ bunch Italian parsley, thick stems removed and washed

3 sprigs fresh oregano, thick stems removed, or 1 teaspoon dried

10 leaves fresh mint, or 1 teaspoon dried

10 leaves fresh basil, or 1 teaspoon dried

1 quart fish stock, home-made preferred

Pinch hot pepper flakes (optional)

1 teaspoon herbal sea salt

1 bunch watercress, thick stems removed and washed

½ pound monkfish, cut into 2-inch pieces

½ pound skinless white fish fillet, such as red snapper, bass, or cod

½ pound regular or rock shrimp, with shells on

1 recipe Bruschetta Italiana (page 50)

2 scallions, cut into 1-inch lengths

Healthful Hint: To help prevent arthritis, you need a wide range of minerals, including copper, selenium, and manganese. While minerals may be depleted from the lands in which we grow our produce, the sea still has an abundant supply, and so do the fish that live there.

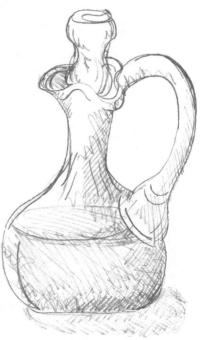

"A little of what you fancy does you good."

—Marie Lloyd

P lace the cleaned mussels and clams in a large bowl of cold water with cornmeal. Add 1 or 2 handfuls of ice and set aside for at least 15 minutes.

In a blender or food processor, pulse mince the onion and garlic. Heat oil in a large stock pot, and add the onion and garlic. Sauté until onion begins to clear, 5 to 7 minutes.

Pulse mince the parsley. Set 2 tablespoons of the parsley aside for the garnish. Pulse mince the oregano, mint, and basil. Add herbs to the onion with the stock, pepper flakes, and salt. Bring to a boil, on a high flame, covered. Lower flame and simmer 10 minutes.

Cut the watercress in 1- to 1½-inch pieces, and set aside.

Add the monkfish and return pot to a boil, covered.

Remove the mussels and clams from the cornmeal water and rinse. Discard water. Add the mussels and clams to the stock pot, cover, and continue cooking on a high flame until the shells open, about 3 to 5 minutes.

Add the white fish fillet (uncut) and shrimp. Continue cooking, covered, on a medium-high flame until the fish is opaque and the shrimp is pink, about 4 or 5 minutes.

Toss watercress into pot. Place a thick trivet on the table and set the pot on it. Scoop a variety of shellfish and fish into individual serving bowls, and ladle broth over these. Sprinkle with scallions and remaining parsley. Serve Bruschetta Italiana (page 50) in a basket for dunking and munching.

YIELD: 4 SERVINGS

NOTE: Mussels can usually be purchased with the beard removed. If you can't find them in this form, scrub the mussels with a brush and, using your hand or a pliers, pull the beard out and discard. (An excellent job for a family member or friend.)

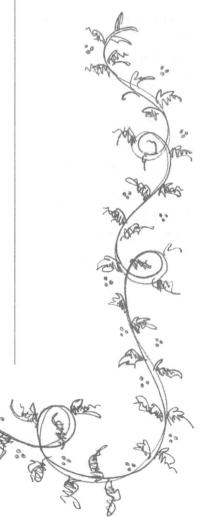

Caldo de Ostiones

This Latin oyster stew is easy to prepare and full of natural flavors. Enjoy this hearty meal with a big wedge of crusty whole grain bread for dunking.

1 pint shucked oysters and juice liquid, about 2 dozen

2 cups fish or chicken stock, homemade preferred

2 garlic cloves, peeled

1 onion, peeled and quartered

1 stalk celery, quartered

4 sprigs fresh parsley, thick stems removed and washed

1 bay leaf

½ teaspoon thyme

1 teaspoon herbal sea salt

¼ teaspoon ground pepper

10 to 12 button mushrooms

2 tablespoons lemon juice

3 scallions, pulse chopped

P lace a fine mesh or cheesecloth-lined sieve over a bowl. Pour the oysters and liquid in. Remove oysters from the sieve into a small bowl, as the liquid is draining. Reserve the liquid.

Rinse oysters, rubbing lightly to loosen grit and sand. In a 4-quart pot, bring the stock to a boil, covered.

In a blender or food processor, pulse mince the garlic, onion, celery, and parsley, and add to the stock with the bay leaf, thyme, herbal salt, and pepper. Stir, and reduce flame and simmer, covered.

Pulse chop the mushrooms and add to the pot. Stir once to mix thoroughly and cook for about 10 minutes.

Add the oysters, reserved oyster liquid, and lemon juice. Heat gently for about 5 more minutes. Do not boil. Discard the bay leaf.

Serve in large, wide bowls and sprinkle with scallions.

YIELD: 4 SERVINGS

HEALTHFUL HINT: Arthritis drugs such as corticosteroids can cause the body to lose zinc, which is essential for overall good health. Oysters are full of zinc and are a great natural way to increase your body's nutrient intake.

"Eat!"
—Mom

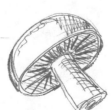

Mediterranean Fillet of Sole Almondine

This traditional almondine recipe has a Mediterranean twist. Easy to prepare and immensely flavorful, this is a dish you'll make again and again.

Wash fillets in cold water and place in a colander to drain.

In a shallow, wide bowl, mix together the flour, garlic, oregano, herbal salt, and pepper. In another shallow bowl, whisk the egg. Dip the sole in egg, and then dust with flour. Place on a clean, dry plate. Continue this process until all the fillets have been floured. Melt 1 tablespoon of ghee or butter in a large skillet over medium-high heat. Add 1 or 2 fillets to skillet. Do not overcrowd. Cook until golden, about 3 minutes. Using a spatula, carefully turn fillets over and cook another 3 minutes, until golden. Add another ½ tablespoon ghee or butter, if needed. Transfer to a warm platter, and cover. Repeat procedure, adding more ghee, until all fillets are cooked.

Coarsely pulse chop the almonds. Melt 1 tablespoon ghee in the skillet. Add almonds and brown lightly, about 2 to 3 minutes. Toss on top of sole.

Garnish fish platter with lemon wedges, and serve immediately.

YIELD: 4 SERVINGS

1 pound skinless fillets of sole or flounder

½ cup whole wheat flour

½ teaspoon garlic powder

½ teaspoon oregano, dried

¼ teaspoon herbal sea salt

Pinch ground pepper

1 egg, organic preferred

4 to 5 tablespoons ghee or unsalted butter

¼ cup raw almonds

1 lemon, cut into wedges

HEALTHFUL HINT: The almonds in the "Almondine" add an extra bit of fat — the good kind, monounsaturates — associated with the healthy heart diet of the Mediterranean. This fat also contains the antioxidant vitamin E.

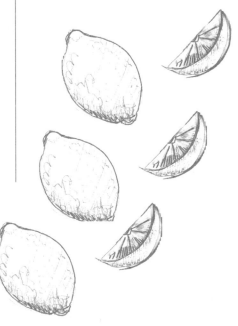

Beef, Pork, and Lamb

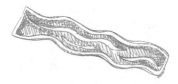

Ossobucco Gremolata

Leg of Lamb Provençale

Stuffed Polish Cabbage

Colorful Steak Fajitas

Grilled Southern Pork Tenderloins

Bring Back Your Mother's Liver 'n Onions!

Royal Mixed Grill

Hearty and Healthy Oxtail Stew

Ossobucco Gremolata

This healthy version of the ever-popular Italian staple for cooking marrow bones. It gets its flavor surge from the combination of savory herbs, spices, and citrus zests.

4 veal shank bones, each about 2 inches thick

½ cup whole wheat flour

½ teaspoon sea salt

¼ teaspoon ground black pepper

2 tablespoons extra virgin olive oil

2 tablespoons unsalted butter or ghee

1 onion, peeled and quartered

2 stalks celery, quartered

10 leaves fresh basil

1 teaspoon rosemary

½ cup dry white wine (optional), or additional stock

1 cup chicken or beef stock, homemade preferred

1 recipe Gremolata (see page 162)

Wash the shanks in cold water and set on a plate to drain slightly. In a wide, shallow bowl, mix the flour, salt, and pepper. Coat the shanks with flour.

Heat an ovenproof medium-size skillet, on a high flame, and add the oil and butter. Place the shanks in the pan upright. Reduce the heat, and cook until the meat on the bones is light brown, turning several times, about 15 minutes.

In a blender or food processor, pulse mince the onion, celery, basil, and rosemary. Add the wine (or additional stock) and stock, and cover. Simmer the shanks on a low heat until the meat is very tender (or bake them, covered, in a preheated 325 degree oven), for 1 hour.

Sprinkle the tops of the bones with the Gremolata, cover, and cook another 5 minutes. Serve hot.

YIELD: 4 SERVINGS

HEALTHFUL HINT: One of the reasons veal shanks are so delicious is the gelatinous marrow within each shank. Boost your gelatin intake to heal worn joints with this classic Italian dish.

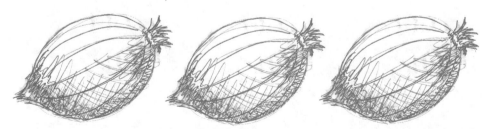

Leg of Lamb Provençale

This very elegant and impressive dish is also quite simple to prepare. It is a lovely presentation for any dinner table.

POSITION THE OVEN SHELVES TO FIT THE LAMB.
PREHEAT THE OVEN TO 450 DEGREES.

I n a small processor, pulse mince the garlic and rosemary. Put in a small bowl, with the mustard and oil. Mix well.

Wash the lamb in cold water and dry with paper toweling. Using a paring knife, remove the fell membrane (papery white outer covering).

Spread the mustard mixture on all sides of the lamb. Place the meat in a roasting pan fitted with a rack, with the fat side up. Put in the oven, and immediately reduce the temperature to 325 degrees.

Roast the lamb 25 minutes to the pound, for meat that is still pink in the center. (For a 5-pound leg of lamb, about 2 hours and 5 minutes.) Adjust the time for taste preferences.

When done, remove the lamb from the oven and let it sit a few minutes before carving. Serve the lamb with pan drippings drained of excess fat, in a gravy boat.

YIELD: 8 SERVINGS

Remove the lamb from the refrigerator about 1 hour before cooking.

4 cloves garlic, peeled

1 tablespoon rosemary

½ cup Dijon mustard

3 tablespoons extra virgin olive oil

One 5-pound leg of lamb

HEALTHFUL HINT: If you have been using steroids and NSAID medications for your arthritis, you may be low in certain nutrients such as iron, phosphorous, and potassium. Meats such as lamb are high in phosphorus and will help replenish your supply.

Stuffed Polish Cabbage

No, this isn't your heavy sour cream, after-polka feast for a gourmand. In fact, this unique dish is quite healthy and light, yet very satisfying.

1 medium cabbage

2½ to 3 quarts boiling puri-fied water

1 onion, peeled and quartered

1 clove garlic, peeled

¼ bunch fresh parsley, thick stems removed and washed (see Note)

¼ bunch fresh dill, thick stems removed and washed

1 pound lean ground beef, organic preferred

2 tablespoons currants or raisins, unsulphured preferred

2 eggs, organic preferred

1 cup whole grain bread crumbs

1 teaspoon sea salt

½ teaspoon ground pepper

One 18-inch piece cheese-cloth

4 cups chicken stock, home-made preferred

1 stalk celery, quartered

1 bay leaf

1 recipe Georgian Yogurt Sauce (page 165)

Using a paring knife, remove the inner core from the cabbage. Put the cabbage in the pot of boiling water. Place a heat-proof plate on top of the cabbage to keep it immersed in the water, and cover the pot. Cook on a high flame, for 5 to 7 minutes. Turn off the flame and uncover.

In a blender or food processor, pulse chop onion, garlic, parsley, and dill, and put it a large bowl. Combine with the beef, currants or raisins, eggs, bread crumbs, salt, and pepper. Mix well.

Using a large slotted spoon and tongs, carefully remove the cabbage from the cooking water, into a large bowl. Cover with cold water, until the cabbage is cool enough to touch. Peel the leaves away, and set them in a colander to drain and cool further.

Position the oven shelves to fit a Dutch oven.

PREHEAT OVEN TO 450 DEGREES.

HEALTHFUL HINT: Vitamin C is full of joint-protecting bioflavonoids, and cabbage and parsley are a great source of it. Fresh herbs, such as the parsley and dill in this recipe, can be found in grocery stores.

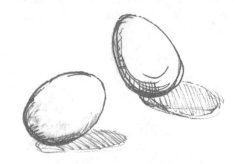

Spread out the cheesecloth and place 3 of the largest cabbage leaves in the center of the cheesecloth. Spread a layer of meat mixture on the leaves. Add 3 more leaves, and more meat, and continue this process until all the leaves and meat mixture are used up, ending with a meat layer.

Pull the corners of the cheesecloth together, wrapping it tightly around the cabbage leaves and stuffing, to form a ball. Tie opposite corners together, enclosing the stuffed cabbage.

Place the stuffed cabbage in the Dutch oven, add stock, celery pieces, and bay leaf. Cover and bake about 1½ hours, basting occasionally.

Using tongs, carefully remove the cabbage ball to a large platter. (Store leftover cooking liquid and use as the base for a rich and flavorful soup.) With a pair of kitchen scissors, cut the cheesecloth away and discard. Cut the cabbage into wedges and serve with Georgian Yogurt Sauce.

YIELD: 4 SERVINGS

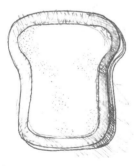

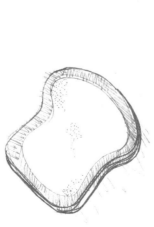

NOTE: If you've purchased a bunch of fresh herbs and there is too much to use over several days, just hang them upside down, and allow the herbs to dry.

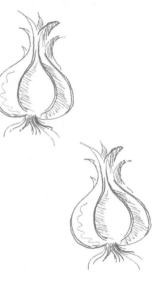

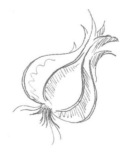

STASH & SNACK

Colorful Steak Fajitas

When you're trying to monitor your diet, the tastier the food the better. Look south of the border for meal inspiration.

Prepare the marinade, and marinate the steak for at least 2 hours.

4 cloves garlic, peeled

¾ cup lime or lemon juice, fresh preferred

6 tablespoons extra virgin olive oil

1 tablespoon imported soy sauce

½ teaspoon ground black pepper

One 1- to 1½ -pound flank steak, trimmed of fat

2 tablespoons unsalted butter

1 onion, peeled and sliced

1 red bell pepper, seeded and sliced

1 green bell pepper, seeded and sliced

2 plum tomatoes, cored and quartered

1 yellow summer squash, sliced

1 teaspoon herbal sea salt

½ bunch cilantro or parsley, pulse chopped

16 corn tortillas, warmed

TO PREPARE THE MARINADE:

In a blender or food processor, puree the garlic. Add the lime or lemon juice, 4 tablespoons oil, soy sauce, and pepper. Pour the marinade into a large, non metallic container with a lid. Add the steak, cover, and marinate for at least 2 hours in the refrigerator. Turn the steak over after 1 hour.

TO PREPARE THE FAJITAS:

When the steak has finished marinating, remove from the marinade, and pat it dry with paper toweling. Strain the remaining marinade and reserve.

Position the oven rack about 3 inches from the broiler heat source. Preheat the broiler.

Broil for about 2 minutes on each side; the outside should be appetizingly charred but the interior should still be rare (so the steak can be later cooked with the marinade without toughening). Turn the broiler off, and proceed with the vegetables, leaving the steak in the oven.

Heat a cast-iron skillet or griddle and add the butter and remaining 2 tablespoons oil, making sure the fat coats the bottom of the skillet evenly.

HEALTHFUL HINT: Red and green peppers, and tomatoes, are particularly high in vitamin C which is an antioxidant known to squash free radicals. Vitamin C is sensitive to heat and is easily destroyed by cooking or processing, so be careful when preparing this dish to keep the vegetables slightly crisp.

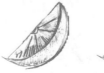

Add the onion, and sauté over a high flame to brown the onion edges, about 3 minutes. Add the red and green peppers, and cook another 3 minutes. Keep the heat high enough to char the vegetables without cooking them all the way through. Add the tomatoes, yellow squash, and salt. Lower heat, and cook for 3 more minutes. The vegetables should still be crisp.

Meanwhile, remove the steak from the oven. Lay it on a cutting board and cut it against the grain into ¼-inch slices. (Do not cut on the diagonal. This would negate the effect of tenderness to be gained by cutting directly against the grain.)

Raise the heat on the griddle to very hot, and add the steak. Drizzle ¼ cup of the reserved marinade onto the steak and vegetables, at little at a time. If the pan is hot enough, the marinade should evaporate upon contact. Do not create a puddle of liquid in the skillet.

Place a trivet on the table, and put the pan on it. Sprinkle with the cilantro or parsley. Serve at once, right from the pan, with warm tortillas and other garnishes.

YIELD: 4 SERVINGS

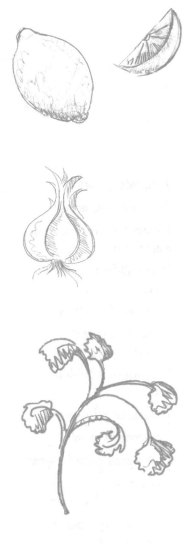

"A complete lack of caution is perhaps one of the true signs of a real gourmet: he has no need for it, being filled as he is with a God-given and intelligently self-cultivated sense of gastronomical freedom."

—M.F.K. Fisher

Grilled Southern Pork Tenderloins

This sweet and sour version of a traditional Southern favorite uses fruits, herbs, and spices to create an unforgettable marinade.

Prepare the marinade and marinate the pork tenderloins for 2 to 4 hours, or overnight.

2 shallots, peeled

2 garlic cloves, peeled

1 walnut-sized knob fresh ginger root

½ cup all-fruit apricot or peach conserves

½ cup purified water

2 tablespoons real vanilla extract

2 tablespoons fresh lemon juice

1 teaspoon dried thyme

1 teaspoon sea salt

½ teaspoon ground pepper

One 1-pound pork tenderloin, cut in 1-inch-thick pieces

½ cup chicken stock, home-made preferred

1 tablespoon unsalted butter

NOTE: To grill: Place the meat on a preheated grill. Cover, making sure the vents are open. Cook for 15 minutes, basting occasionally. Turn meat over and grill until the internal temperature is 160 degrees, about another 10 minutes. Remove from the grill and slice.

TO PREPARE THE MARINADE: In a blender or food processor, pulse mince the shallots, garlic, and ginger. Put into a small bowl with the conserves, water, vanilla, lemon juice, thyme, salt, and pepper.

Arrange pork in a large, shallow, nonmetallic dish, and pour the apricot marinade over. Turn to coat evenly. Cover and refrigerate for 2 to 4 hours.

TO COOK THE PORK: Position the oven rack about 3 inches from the broiler heat source. Preheat the broiler or prepare the grill (see Note).

Remove the pork from the marinade and shake slightly, allowing excess marinade to drip off. Reserve marinade. Place pork on a broiler rack, and slide under the broiler. Sear on each side for about 2 minutes.

Baste the tenderloins with the remaining marinade. Close the oven door and change the setting to bake, with the temperature at 375 degrees. Bake for 20 to 25 minutes.

Meanwhile, place the remaining marinade in a small sauce pan and add stock and butter. Bring to a boil, uncovered, reduce heat and simmer about 5 minutes. Taste and add additional salt and pepper, if desired.

Arrange on a platter. Drizzle sauce over, and serve.

YIELD: 4 SERVINGS

HEALTHFUL HINT: Pork tenderloin is actually considered a very lean and healthy mea and provides a wide range of vitamins and minerals. Make sure it's cooked thoroughly, with no pink in the center. Fresh ginger helps aid the digestion of pork and adds a spicy-sweet fla vor, perking up the marinade.

Bring Back Your Mother's Liver 'n Onions!

A good, organic cut of liver, cooked to perfection, is actually quite tasty and is full of vitamins and minerals. Your mother knew what she was doing when she served this dish.

S lice or pulse chop the onions. Heat a skillet on a medium-high flame, and melt 2 tablespoons butter. Add the onions and cook until they begin to brown, about 10 minutes.

Push the onions to the side of pan, making room to add liver. Add remaining 1 tablespoon butter. Place liver on top of the butter, and sprinkle with salt and pepper. Cook liver for 2 to 3 minutes.

Turn the liver over, and season again with salt and pepper. With a spoon, push the onions on top of the liver, while cooking another 2 to 3 minutes. Serve immediately, with a side of Russian Mushroom Kasha.

YIELD: 4 SERVINGS

EALTHFUL HINT: Liver is extraordinarily high in vitamins and minerals, such as vitamins A, K, B12, and C, and niacin, folic acid, copper, selenium, iron, and zinc—a very rich source of those nutrients that soothe painful joints and inflammation.

3 onions, peeled

3 tablespoons unsalted butter

¾ to 1 pound organic calf's liver

Sea salt

Ground pepper

1 recipe Russian Mushroom Kasha (page 59)

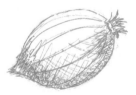

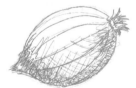

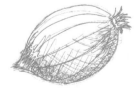

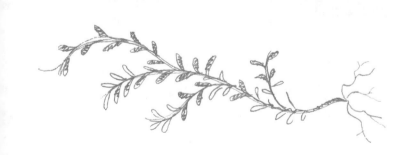

Royal Mixed Grill

This classic dish is a quick fix that spares sore joints. Yes, the Mixed Grill comes with calories, but don't avoid this savory dish—just have smaller portions.

2 organic chicken livers (see Note)

2 slices nitrite-free bacon

4 lamb chops

2 link sausages, organic preferred

8 mushroom caps

2 tomatoes

Extra virgin olive oil

Herbal sea salt

Ground pepper

NOTE: If you can't find organic liver and nitrite-fee bacon, leave them out of this recipe.

Position the oven rack about 3 inches from the broiler heat source. Preheat the broiler.

Cut the livers and bacon slices in half. Wrap a half a slice of bacon around each liver and secure it with a wooden toothpick. Place them on a broiler pan fitted with a rack, along with the chops and sausages.

Put the mushrooms on a heat-proof plate and drizzle with a little oil, and sprinkle with salt and pepper.

Cut the tomatoes in half. Place on the same plate with the mushrooms and season with oil, salt, and pepper. Place the plate on the rack with the meats.

Slide the rack under the broiler, and cook for 2 minutes. Turn the livers and mushrooms, and cook another 2 minutes. Do not turn the tomatoes.

Remove the livers, mushrooms, and tomatoes to a platter, and cover. Turn the chops and sausages, and cook another 3 to 5 minutes.

Remove the chops and sausages to the platter. Serve immediately.

YIELD: 4 SERVINGS

HEALTHFUL HINT: Animal foods such as the lamb and sausages provide a good source of vitamin A, one of the antioxidants. Organ meats such as liver provide iron which counteract the iron loss that can be caused by taking NSAIDs.

Hearty and Healthy Oxtail Stew

Open yourself to trying some old-fashioned recipes such as this delicious stew that features well-simmered bones. Once considered the food of poor people, this gourmet, gelatin-rich stew will soothe your joints while your taste buds dance!

POSITION THE OVEN SHELVES TO FIT THE DUTCH OVEN.
PREHEAT THE OVEN TO 350 DEGREES.

Wash the oxtails in cold water, and pat dry. Melt the butter or ghee in a Dutch oven, on a medium-high heat. Add the oxtails. Cook until brown, turning on all sides, about 10 minutes.

Add the stock, vinegar, bay leaf, thyme, salt, and pepper, and bring to a boil.

Cover the pot and place in the oven. Cook until tender, about 2 to 3 hours. Using tongs, turn the bones over after 1 hour.

In a blender or food processor, pulse chop the carrot, celery, turnip, onion, and garlic. Add to the oxtails after 1½ hours of cooking. Add more stock or water, if needed, and return to the oven.

When meat is very tender, remove the oxtails to a deep platter and cover to keep them warm. Using a colander set into a nonplastic bowl, strain the cooking liquid. Return the liquid to the pot, and set the vegetables aside.

Using a whisk, blend the flour into the cooking liquid. Heat to a boil over medium flame. Continue whisking until the mixture has thickened to a gravy. Add more stock or water to thin, if needed. Taste and adjust seasoning, if desired.

With the flame still on, return the oxtails and vegetables to the gravy. Mix well. Serve hot, over noodles.

YIELD: 4 SERVINGS

8 to 12 oxtail joints (see Note)

¼ cup unsalted butter or ghee

3 cups beef stock, homemade preferred

1 teaspoon cider vinegar

1 bay leaf

½ teaspoon dried thyme

1 teaspoon sea salt

½ teaspoon ground pepper

2 carrots, trimmed and quartered

2 ribs celery, quartered

2 turnips, trimmed and quartered

1 onion, peeled and quartered

2 garlic cloves, peeled

2 tablespoons whole wheat flour

Cooked whole wheat noodles

NOTE: If the joints do not come already separated, have your butcher do this for you.

HEALTHFUL HINT: Gelatin is a balm to arthritic joints; and bones, when cooked, release gelatin and nutritious minerals.

Sauces and Toppings

Sweet Red Pepper Sauce

Papaya-Mango Salsa

Gremolata

Perfect Pesto

Satay Sauce

Georgian Yogurt Sauce

Garlic-Onion Jam

Ginger Root Chutney

Sun-dried Tomato Mayonnaise

Whipped Strawberry Sauce

Creamy Fruit Topping

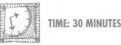

Sweet Red Pepper Sauce

This aromatic roasted pepper sauce is a great spread for breads, and offers an excellent flavor to broiled meats, vegetables, and whole grain pastas.

3 large sweet red peppers

2 cloves garlic, peeled

1 tablespoon to ¼ cup extra virgin olive oil

2 tablespoons whole grain bread crumbs

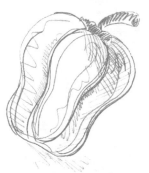

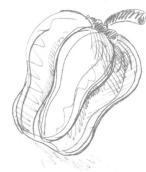

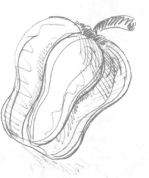

PREHEAT THE BROILER.

Place the peppers on an ungreased baking sheet. Put them under the broiler for 10 to 15 minutes, turning the pepper several times. They will become soft, and the skins will char and wrinkle.

Place the peppers in a paper bag and close the top, or drop into a bowl and cover. Allow to cool, about 10 minutes.

Rubbing the skins with your fingers, peel off and remove the skin; discard. Using a plate to catch the liquid, cut the peppers in half and remove the seeds.

In a blender or food processor, place peppers, their juices, and garlic, and puree until smooth.

While the blender or processor is running, carefully drizzle the oil in a thin, steady stream. The mixture will have the consistency of mayonnaise.

Transfer to a medium bowl. Add bread crumbs and mix well.

Refrigerate until ready to use. It will thicken as it sits.

YIELD: 2 CUPS

HEALTHFUL HINT: Sweet peppers have even more vitamin C than oranges, and this vitamin is not only an antioxidant, it also helps maintain connective tissue. You get the most vitamin C benefits when you eat these peppers raw.

Papaya-Mango Salsa

Keep tasty condiments on hand to dress up nutritious cuts of meat and fish. You'll be glad to have this salsa when you need to be a short-order chef.

Cut the papaya in half, and remove and discard the seeds. Using a paring knife, score the flesh in a 1/2-inch crosshatched pattern, being careful not to cut through the skin. Use a spoon and scoop the papaya pieces into a medium bowl. Discard the skin.

Place the mango on a plate to catch the juice. Hold it upright and cut around the mango pit, in thick slices. Score the flesh in a crosshatched pattern, being careful not to cut through the skin. Using a spoon, scoop the mango into the bowl with the papaya. Pour the juices on the plate into the bowl. Discard the skin.

In a small processor, mince the mint and garlic. Add to the fruit with the vinegar, lemon juice, and salt. Stir well. (If the fruit doesn't have enough sweetness for you, add several tablespoons of peach or apricot all-fruit conserves, or honey.)

Store in a covered container and refrigerate until ready to serve.

YIELD: 2¹/₂ CUPS

1 papaya (see Note)

1 mango

5 leaves fresh mint, or ½ teaspoon dried mint

1 garlic clove, peeled

1 tablespoon cider vinegar

1 tablespoon lemon juice

Pinch sea salt

NOTE: If fresh papaya and mangoes are not in season, purchase your favorite unsulphured dry fruit, without sugar. Put ½ cup of each fruit in a small saucepan, add purified water, and bring to a boil, covered. Lower flame and simmer for 3 to 4 minutes. Turn off flame and allow the fruit to rehydrate and cool.

EALTHFUL HINT: Papaya and mint are helpful to the digestion, which when working roperly will better absorb arthritis-protective nutrients.

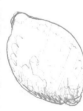
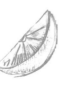
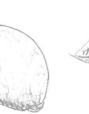
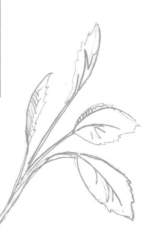

Gremolata

This seasoning mixture is a great way to accent a dish, without using salt.

2 cloves garlic, peeled

4 sprigs fresh parsley, thick stems removed and washed

1 teaspoon grated lemon rind, organic preferred (see Note)

1 teaspoon grated orange rind, organic preferred

NOTE: The skins of organic lemons are free of anti-mold agents and other chemicals, and they taste better.

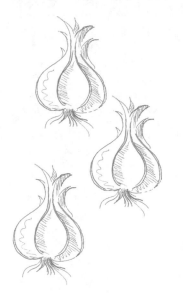

Place the garlic and parsley in a small processor, and finely mince. Add the lemon and orange rinds, mixing briefly.

Sprinkle this mixture on sauce or gravy during the last 5 minutes of cooking. Simmer, covered, over low heat to allow the flavors to absorb.

Store in a covered container in the refrigerator, until ready to use.

YIELD: ¼ CUP

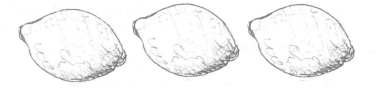

> "So many sauces, so little time."
>
> —David Dortman

Perfect Pesto

Pesto is a classic Italian recipe that has found its way into American cuisine —
and our hearts. It depends on nuts and aged cheese for its richness and depth —
a time-honored condiment with beneficial nutrition. Today, we use it to top off
pasta, as a marinade for meat, to flavor beans, and even as a salad dressing.

In a blender or food processor, finely mince the basil,
cheese, nuts, garlic, and salt. Using a rubber spatula,
scrape the sides of the container.

With the motor running, drizzle in the oils through
the opening in the lid.

Store in a covered glass jar, with a thin layer of olive
oil covering the pesto to keep it from turning black. It
will last in the refrigerator for several months, and in the
freezer for a year (see Note).

YIELD: 3 CUPS

**2 bunches fresh basil, leaves
only, washed (about 4 cups,
packed)**

**¾ cup grated Parmesan
cheese**

¼ cup pignoli or walnuts

4 garlic cloves, peeled

½ teaspoon sea salt

**6 tablespoons extra virgin
olive oil**

2 tablespoons flaxseed oil

NOTE: It is hard to make pesto in
small portions. We suggest you refrigerate the extra for later use or freeze
it. Pack the pesto into the compart-
ments of an ice cube tray. Cover with
plastic film and put into the freezer.
Just pop a cube out when a burst of
flavor is needed. It defrosts quickly.

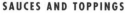

Satay Sauce

Be experimental in your food choices. Here's a brilliant sauce from Thailand, destined to become a staple once you've tried it; it's an exotic way to follow our plan to "eat a variety of foods."

1 onion, peeled and quartered

1 garlic clove, peeled

1 tablespoon unsalted butter or ghee

1 teaspoon ground coriander

½ teaspoon ground cumin

1 teaspoon ground pepper

Pinch red pepper flakes (optional)

½ cup raw almond butter

¾ cup coconut milk (see Note)

2 tablespoons honey or real maple syrup

1 tablespoon fresh lemon or lime juice

1 tablespoon imported soy sauce

Pinch sea salt

NOTE: Coconut milk is available canned. There are several brands that have no added sugar, chemicals, or preservatives. If this type is not available, substitute with purified water and 2 tablespoon unsalted butter. The thick richness of coconut milk is full of potassium and magnesium—nutrients that are good for you, and fine when used in moderation.

In a blender or food processor, pulse mince the onion and garlic.

Heat the butter over moderate heat in a medium-sized skillet. Add the onion-garlic mixture, coriander, cumin, pepper, and pepper flakes. Reduce heat and cook, stirring occasionally, about 5 minutes.

In the blender or food processor, combine the almond butter and ¼ cup coconut milk. Puree until smooth. Add the remaining coconut milk, honey or maple syrup, lemon or lime juice, soy sauce, and salt. Mix well.

Add the almond mixture to the skillet. Cook, uncovered, over low heat, until the sauce is thickened, stirring occasionally, about 15 minutes. Do not let it boil.

Use this sauce hot, warm, room temperature, or cold. Store in a covered container in the refrigerator.

YIELD: ABOUT 1¼ CUPS

HEALTHFUL HINT: We substituted the peanuts that are often used in this sauce with almonds, since almonds contain boron, a needed mineral that is missing in most American meals. Boron is important in maintaining joint health. And it is worthy to note that peanut oil has been seen to cause severe atherosclerosis in laboratory animals. That's enough to keep us away from peanuts in general.

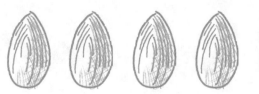

Georgian Yogurt Sauce

This sauce comes from the hills of the former USSR, and is a real find. We use it over pasta, yams, grains, and mixed into beans. There's no end to its versatility; it will become a favorite of yours, too.

I n a small processor, finely mince the garlic. Place in a small bowl with the yogurt, oil, and salt. Mix well. Store in a covered container in the refrigerator, until ready to use.

YIELD: 1 CUP

4 garlic cloves, peeled

1 cup plain yogurt with active cultures

1 tablespoon extra virgin olive oil

¼ teaspoon herbal sea salt

HEALTHFUL HINT: Fermented milk in any of its natural forms—yogurt, kefir, buttermilk, leben, kourmiss, or acidophilus milk—is known to contain "active cultures" that add beneficial bacteria to the intestines. Not all fermented milks are created the same, so purchase one that contains L. acidophilus, L. bulgaricus, and bifidus cultures.

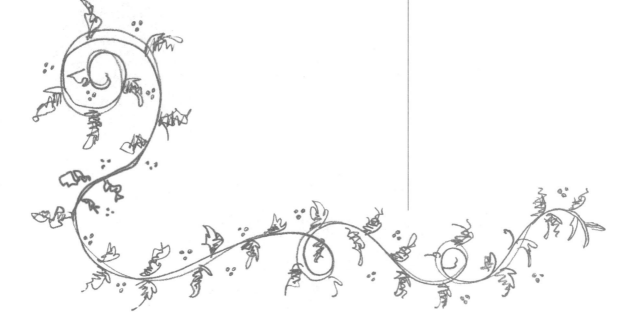

Garlic-Onion Jam

Just toss the garlic and onions in the oven and let the heat do its work. After you've tasted this once—you'll begin using it on everything.

3 onions, unpeeled

1 bulb garlic, unpeeled

2 tablespoons extra virgin olive oil

¼ teaspoon cider vinegar or lemon juice

Pinch cayenne pepper

⅛ teaspoon herbal sea salt

PREHEAT THE OVEN TO 350 DEGREES.

Place the onions and garlic in a Dutch oven. Brush the skins with the oil. Cover and bake until the onions and garlic are very soft when pierced with a sharp knife, about 1 hour.

Remove from the oven and cool.

Squeeze the cloves of garlic and onions from their skins, and place in a blender or food processor. Add the vinegar, cayenne, and salt. Blend until smooth.

YIELD: 1 CUP

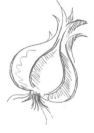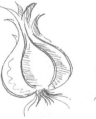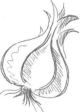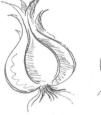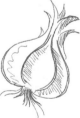

Ginger Root Chutney

Once only seen in Indian cuisine, chutneys are making quite a statement in today's American diet. As a low-fat, high-taste way to add excitement to almost any meal, consider using chutney as an accompaniment.

Wash the ginger, and cut in chunks. In a blender or food processor, mince the ginger finely.

Add the currants, blending again. Using a rubber spatula, scrape the sides of the bowl. Add water, if needed, 1 tablespoon at a time, until a thick paste is formed.

Remove to a small covered container and refrigerate until ready to use.

YIELD: 1 CUP

One 6- to 8-inch piece fresh ginger root, about 4 ounces (see Note)

½ cup currants, unsulphured preferred

Purified water, as needed

NOTE: Young ginger is preferred, with its skin barely formed and still pink. If this is not available, peel the ginger.

HEALTHFUL HINT: This chutney is a way to get extra amounts of arthritis-fighting ginger root, which is also beneficial to the digestion, and is especially useful when eaten with protein foods or beans. And currants are known for their bioflavonoids, which slow inflammation and are also essential for the proper absorption and use of vitamin C, which in turn, allows our bodies to make collagen and connective tissue.

Sun-dried Tomato Mayonnaise

There's nothing tastier than homemade mayo—and this one is missing the sugars and other ingredients found in the commercial ones.

½ cup reconstituted or oil-packed sun-dried tomatoes, unsulphured preferred, drained

1 clove garlic, peeled

¼ cup plain yogurt with active cultures

3 tablespoons extra virgin olive oil or flaxseed oil

1 teaspoon balsamic vinegar or lemon juice

¼ teaspoon sea salt

In a blender or food processor, puree the tomatoes, garlic, and yogurt. Drizzle in the oil while the motor is running, until the mixture thickens slightly. Add the vinegar and salt, and combine well.

YIELD: 1 CUP

HEALTHFUL HINT: Yogurt provides calcium, vitamin D, protein, and other nutrients important for growth and maintenance of strong bones and connective tissues.

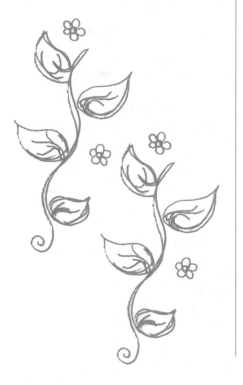

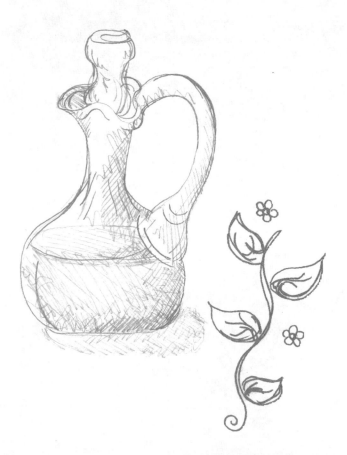

Whipped Strawberry Sauce

Don't limit yourself to using this sauce only on Sunday mornings—add this delectable sweet to yogurt, spread it on toast, smear it on muffins, or add a dollop to hot cereal. You may just want some on a spoon!

Put the strawberries, juice, conserves, and salt in a small pot. Cover and bring to a boil. Reduce flame and simmer until the strawberries are completely cooked, about 10 minutes.

Add the vanilla and cook another minute, uncovered. Turn off flame, stir in the butter, and set aside to cool slightly.

In a blender or food processor, puree the strawberry mixture.

YIELD: 2 CUPS

HEALTHFUL HINT: Strawberries are high in vitamin C and bioflavonoids, as are most berries. Vitamin C is an antioxidant—a free-radical antidote. Bioflavonoids are essential for healthy capillary walls and the metabolism of vitamin C.

1 pint fresh strawberries, washed, stems and leaves removed (see Note)

½ cup unsweetened apple juice

¼ cup all-fruit strawberry conserves

Pinch sea salt

1 teaspoon real vanilla extract

3 tablespoons unsalted butter

NOTE: Substitute the strawberries with raspberries, peaches, blueberries, or any other favorite fruit, and a corresponding all-fruit jam.

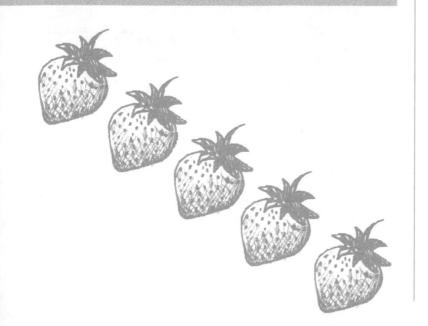

Creamy Fruit Topping

This decadent-tasting yet delicious fruit topping can accompany breakfast dishes such as waffles or pancakes, or can top off any one of our healthy desserts. (We have been seen scooping this topping into a bowl and munching on it with a sprinkling of chopped walnuts!)

1 cup plain yogurt with active cultures

1 banana, quartered

3 tablespoons real maple syrup

¼ teaspoon cinnamon

Favorite fresh fruit or all-fruit conserves (optional)

In a blender or food processor, combine the yogurt, banana, syrup, and cinnamon.

If desired, blend in additional fruit or all-fruit conserves, to change the flavor. Or spoon over berries for an easy and satisfying treat.

Store in a covered container and refrigerate until ready to use.

YIELD: 2½ CUPS

HEALTHFUL HINT: A little fat will satiate your appetite much quicker—keeping you from overeating and consuming excess calories. This creamy topping is full of satisfaction and great taste.

Fruit Desserts and other Treats

Vermont Maple Apple Crisp

Always Delicious Poached Pears

Baked Apple Stuffed with Ginger Root Chutney

Fresh Fruit Aspic

Lemon Sesame Cookies

Hindi Ginger Cookies

Saucy Apple Loaf

No-Bake Cheesy Ricotta Cake

Harvest Season Pie

Influential Greek Rice Pudding

Better Than Any Other Low-Fat Chocolate Brownies!

Vermont Maple Apple Crisp

This classic dessert takes its inspiration from Vermont's fall harvest season, when the apples are ripe.

9 apples of three different varieties such as McIntosh, Red or Golden Delicious, Granny Smith

½ cup real maple syrup

½ cup walnuts, coarsely pulse chopped

¼ cup currants or raisins, unsulphured preferred

½ cup plus 2 tablespoons whole wheat pastry flour

½ teaspoon cinnamon

2 pinches sea salt

4 tablespoons unsalted butter

½ cup rolled oats

1 recipe Creamy Fruit Topping (page 170)

PREHEAT OVEN TO 375 DEGREES. GREASE A 9- X 13-INCH BAKING DISH.

Quarter and core the apples, and cut into chunks or slices. Place in a medium bowl with ¼ cup syrup, walnuts, currants, 2 tablespoons flour, ¼ teaspoon cinnamon, and 1 pinch salt. Mix together and pour into the baking dish.

In a small pot, on a low flame, melt the butter. Turn off the flame. Using a wooden spoon mix in ¼ cup syrup. Add the oats, ½ cup flour, ¼ teaspoon cinnamon, and 1 pinch salt. It will be the consistency of very coarse meal.

Crumble oat mixture over the top of the apples.

Bake until the apples are tender and topping is golden brown, about 45 minutes. Cool 5 minutes before scooping into bowls with a hearty dollop of our Creamy Fruit Topping.

YIELD: 8 SERVINGS

HEALTHFUL HINT: The standard American diet is low in boron since it's not contained in some of our most popular foods such as orange juice, lettuce, and tomatoes. Nuts and apples are high in boron, which is important for joint health, and since this recipe has both of these, it's also good for you.

"Happiness is a habit— cultivate it."
—Elbert Hubbard

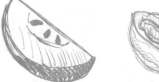

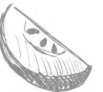

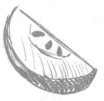

Always Delicious Poached Pears

This is a low-fat dessert with elegance. It's an easy way to get in your quota of fresh fruit—and satisfy your sweet tooth, at the same time.

I n a medium-sized saucepan, combine the juice, syrup, cinnamon, and vanilla. Bring to a boil on a medium flame.

Cut the pears in quarters and core. Add the pears to the saucepan, reduce flame and simmer, covered, until pears are tender, about 15 minutes.

Using a slotted spoon, remove the fruit to a serving bowl. Boil the liquid, uncovered, until it is slightly thickened and reduced, about 10 minutes.

Discard the cinnamon stick. Pour the fruit syrup over the pears and set aside to cool.

In a small bowl, add the yogurt, pinch sea salt, and mix with enough of the syrup to thin and to sweeten to your tastes.

Place 3 pear quarters in each individual serving bowl, with some syrup. Spoon the yogurt sauce over and grate a little fresh nutmeg on top.

YIELD: 4 SERVINGS

1 cup unsweetened apple juice

¼ cup real maple syrup

1 cinnamon stick

I teaspoon real vanilla extract

3 Bosc pears

1 cup plain yogurt with active cultures

Pinch sea salt

Nutmeg

HEALTHY HINT: We use real maple syrup in our recipes because it contains some vitamins and minerals, instead of robbing them from your bones, as sugar does.

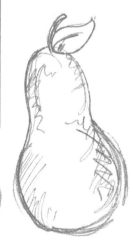

Baked Apple Stuffed with Ginger Root Chutney

Full of flavor, warming for the soul, delicious to the taste buds, helpful for the joints, fast to make, simple ingredients to have or buy—we could go on, but we think you've got the picture. Don't pass this one up!

4 apples, choose your favorite variety

1 recipe Ginger Root Chutney (page 167)

1 cup unsweetened apple juice

PREHEAT THE OVEN TO 350 DEGREES.

Using an apple corer or melon baller, carefully remove the apple core, leaving a ½ inch unremoved on the bottom of the hole. (Do not go through the bottom of the apple.) Using a paring knife, score the apple around the diameter.

Stuff the apples with the Ginger Root Chutney, and place in a baking dish. Pour the juice into the dish.

Bake uncovered, until the apples are soft when pierced with a paring knife, 35 to 40 minutes.

Remove from the oven and serve with several spoonfuls of juice basted over the top.

YIELD: 4 SERVINGS

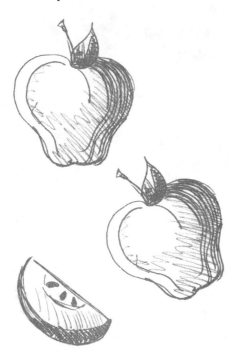

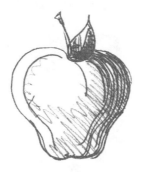

Fresh Fruit Aspic

This easy-to-prepare dessert combines healthy fruit juices with joint-enhancing gelatin. We suggest using a mixture of juices, such as apple and orange juice, or pineapple and apricot juice, or try one of the many sugar-free flavor combinations that are available.

I n a medium-size saucepan, pour in ½ cup cold juice, sprinkle the gelatin over, and stir. Heat on a medium flame and stir constantly, until the gelatin is completely dissolved, about 3 to 5 minutes. Add vanilla and cook another 30 seconds.

Remove from the heat, and stir in the remaining juice. Add the fresh fruit, and stir to cover with the juice. Pour into 4 individual goblets or a single mold. Chill until set.

YIELD: 4 SERVINGS

2 cups unsweetened fruit juice of your choice

1 envelope unflavored gelatin (see Note)

1 teaspoon real vanilla extract

1 cup mixed fresh fruit such as any berries, peaches, bananas, and grapes, sliced

HEALTHFUL HINT: Packaged gelatin desserts have lots of refined sugar with empty calories—and they have no vitamins or minerals. And gelatin is a balm to arthritic joints. Try this healthy alternative instead.

NOTE: Unflavored gelatin, made from animal sources, is widely available and gives consistent results. Agar, a seaweed derivative, is available in natural food stores and offers a vegetarian alternative.

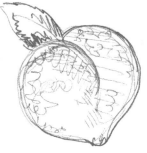
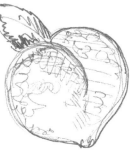
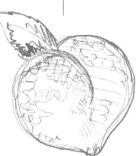
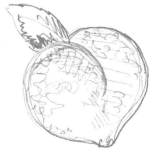

Lemon Sesame Cookies

Unhulled sesame seeds are high in calcium and essential minerals. In this recipe they add a wonderful nutty taste and a crunchy texture.

½ cup unsalted butter, room temperature

1 cup real maple syrup or honey

Zest of 2 lemons, organic preferred

½ cup fresh lemon juice

1 egg, organic preferred

1 tablespoon real vanilla extract

½ teaspoon sea salt

½ cup unhulled sesame seeds

2 cups whole wheat pastry flour

½ cup oatmeal

2 teaspoons baking powder

PREHEAT THE OVEN TO 350 DEGREES.
PREPARE 2 OR 3 COOKIE SHEETS WITH PARCHMENT PAPER, OR GREASE WITH BUTTER.

In a medium bowl or food processor, beat the butter until smooth and soft. Add the maple syrup, lemon zest and juice, egg, vanilla, and salt. Beat well to combine.

In a heavy bottomed skillet, lightly toast the sesame seeds, stirring constantly, about 5 minutes. Some will pop out of the pan. Remove from the skillet as soon as they are toasted to prevent scorching.

In a large bowl, combine the flour, sesame seeds, oatmeal, and baking powder. Add the butter mixture to the flour and stir until moistened.

Drop teaspoonsful of cookie dough onto the prepared sheets, allowing room for the cookies to spread. Bake until the edges turn golden brown, about 10 to 12 minutes.

Using a metal spatula, remove the cookies to a cooling rack. Store in a covered jar.

YIELD: 2 DOZEN COOKIES

HEALTHFUL HINT: Seeds and nuts are full of essential fats that are good for us, and these fats can also go rancid quickly. To avoid rancidity buy only whole, unroasted, raw seeds and nuts, and keep them refrigerated.

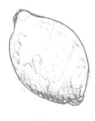
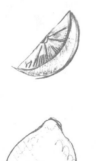
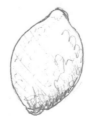

THE ARTHRITIS CURE COOKBOOK

Hindi Ginger Cookies

These spicy ginger cookies make a perfect afternoon snack. You can be sure your family will enjoy them too

PREHEAT OVEN TO 350 DEGREES.
PREPARE TWO COOKIE SHEETS WITH PARCHMENT PAPER, OR GREASE WITH BUTTER.

In a blender or food processor, combine the molasses, butter, baking soda, hot water, ginger, and cinnamon. Add ½ cup flour at a time, to make a firm dough.

On a very lightly floured surface, roll the dough out and cut into shapes with a cookie cutter. Place on the baking sheet.

Bake until golden, about 10 minutes. Cool on a rack.

YIELD: 2 DOZEN

½ cup unsulphured blackstrap molasses

1 tablespoon unsalted butter

½ teaspoon baking soda

1 teaspoon hot purified water

1½ teaspoons ground ginger

½ teaspoon ground cinnamon

1¾ cups whole wheat pastry flour

HEALTHFUL HINT: Ginger has been used for thousands of years in Ayurvedic medicine—India's system of traditional healing—to treat various musculoskeletal diseases and to relieve morning aches and stiffness caused by arthritic joints.

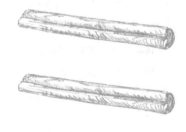

"Civilization has taught us to eat with a fork, but even now if nobody is around we use our fingers."

—Will Rogers

Saucy Apple Loaf

This tasty cake features nutrient-rich molasses instead of refined sugar. Because of its rich taste, the recipe uses a lesser amount of sweetener. Uneaten slices freeze well and make a great on-the-go breakfast.

¼ cup unsalted butter plus extra to grease the pan, at room temperature

½ cup unsulphured black-strap molasses

¼ cup real maple syrup or honey

1 egg, organic preferred

1 cup unsweetened apple-sauce

2 tablespoons lemon juice

1 teaspoon cinnamon

¾ teaspoon baking soda

¼ teaspoon sea salt

½ cup raisins, unsulphured preferred

1 ½ cups whole wheat pastry flour

PREHEAT OVEN TO 350 DEGREES.
GREASE AND FLOUR AN 8-INCH LOAF PAN.

Using an electric mixer or food processor, beat the butter until smooth and soft. Add the molasses, syrup or honey, egg, applesauce, lemon juice, cinnamon, soda, and salt. Mix well.

In a small bowl, mix the raisins with a little flour, and add, along with the remaining flour, to the butter mixture. Stir just enough to moisten and form a smooth batter. Pour into the loaf pan, and bake until firm, about 1 hour.

Remove the loaf from the oven and cool in the pan for 10 minutes. Transfer to a cooling rack, and cool completely before serving.

YIELD: ONE 8-INCH LOAF

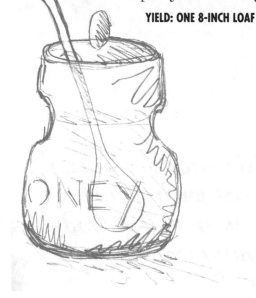

No-Bake Cheesy Ricotta Cake

With this tasty recipe, we've woven beneficial gelatin into a meal, which is not only beneficial to your joints, but adds a updated twist to this perennial favorite.

In a blender or food processor, grind the almonds or sunflower seeds into a meal. Add the cookie or cracker crumbs, almond butter, honey, and pinch salt, and combine well. With wet fingers, press the mixture into the bottom of a 9-inch springform pan. Chill.

In a blender, beat the eggs with the yogurt or buttermilk and ¼ teaspoon salt. Pour into a medium saucepan.

Sprinkle gelatin on yogurt mixture and combine. Place over low heat and cook, stirring constantly, until gelatin dissolves and mixture thickens slightly. Do not boil.

In a blender or food processor, beat the ricotta until smooth and light. Add honey, lemon juice, zest, and vanilla. Add the gelatin mixture and stir until evenly blended. Stir in the dates.

Pour into the chilled crust. Return to the refrigerator and chill for several hours until firm.

Soften conserves by stirring. Spread a layer over the top of the cake.

To serve, slide a paring knife around the edges of the pan, release the spring, and remove side. Place on a cake plate and voilà! (See Note.)

YIELD: ONE 9-INCH CAKE

NOTE: You can garnish the top of the cake with unsweetened coconut flakes, or Whipped Strawberry Sauce (page 169) topped with sliced fresh fruit.

½ cup raw almond or sunflower seeds

½ cup whole grain cookies or cracker crumbs

2 tablespoons raw almond butter

1 tablespoon honey or real maple syrup

Pinch plus ¼ teaspoon salt

4 eggs, organic preferred

1 ¼ cups plain yogurt or buttermilk with active cultures

2 envelopes unflavored gelatin

4 cups ricotta cheese

½ cup honey or maple syrup

1 tablespoon lemon juice

1 teaspoon grated lemon or orange zest, organic preferred

1 teaspoon real vanilla extract

½ cup chopped dates

½ cup all-fruit raspberry conserves

Harvest Season Pie

Pour this yummy filling into a pre-baked pie shell, and a gourmet dessert will be ready in no time at all. Or forget the pie shell and scoop it into champagne glasses, for a wonderful treat.

This recipe requires a pre-baked pie crust (see Note).

6 apples, quartered and cored

12 pitted dates

3 tablespoons unsalted butter

1 teaspoon ground cinnamon

½ teaspoon ground ginger

¼ teaspoon ground nutmeg

Pinch sea salt

1 pre-baked whole wheat pie crust

½ cup raw or toasted walnut pieces

NOTE: You can find whole wheat pie shells in the freezer section in a natural food store. We keep several sets in the freezer. If these are not available, spoon into individual goblets and then top with walnuts.

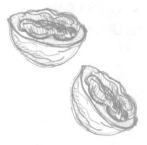

I n a blender or food processor, chop the apples into small chunks. Put in a medium saucepan. Put the dates in processor and chop into small bits. Add to the apples with the butter, cinnamon, ginger, nutmeg, and salt. Toss together.

Cover and cook on a medium-low flame until the apples are tender but not mushy, about 8 to 10 minutes. Stir once or twice during cooking.

Spoon the filling into the baked shell, if you wish to eat it warm. Or let the filling cool to room temperature and spoon it into the pie shell just before serving to keep the crust from getting soggy. Top with walnuts.

YIELD: 1 PIE

HEALTHFUL HINT: The cinnamon and ginger in this dessert reduce inflammation, and the sweetness in this recipe come from nutritious natural fruit sugars.

"If this was adulthood, the only improvement she could detect in her situation was that now she could eat dessert without eating her vegetables."

—Lisa Alther, *Other Women*

Influential Greek Rice Pudding

This very flavorful pudding is a healthy dessert and a great alternative to packaged puddings. With the addition of the cooked rice, it is infinitely more nutritious.

I n a medium saucepan, combine the cooked rice, eggs, yogurt or buttermilk, maple syrup, cinnamon, nutmeg, currants, and salt.

Cook over medium heat, stirring constantly, until thick, about 10 to 15 minutes. Do not boil. (If desired, cook the pudding in the top of a double boiler. Stir occasionally. This method takes about 30 minutes, but requires less attention.)

Stir in vanilla, and cook another 30 seconds.

Pour into a ceramic serving bowl or individual goblets and serve warm. Or cover and chill.

YIELD: 6 SERVINGS

HEALTHFUL HINT: Don't make this recipe with white rice. You'll short-change yourself of the vitamins and minerals your body and joints need. Brown rice is a great source of vitamin E and selenium, critical antioxidants, while white rice has virtually none.

This recipe requires pre-cooked brown rice.

2 cups cooked brown rice

2 eggs, organic preferred, lightly beaten

2 cups plain yogurt or buttermilk with active cultures

⅓ cup real maple syrup

½ teaspoon ground cinnamon

½ teaspoon ground nutmeg

¼ cup currants, unsulphured preferred

Pinch sea salt

1 teaspoon real vanilla extract

TIME: 45 MINUTES

Better Than Any Other Low-Fat Chocolate Brownies!

Most people steer clear of brownies when monitoring their diet. And generally, the low-fat alternatives are also low in taste. Not this brownie. Moist and flavorful, this is one dessert that you won't have to feel guilty about.

⅓ cup unsweetened cocoa powder

½ cup whole wheat pastry flour

¼ teaspoon sea salt

½ cup real maple syrup

½ cup pureed prunes (see Note)

½ cup chopped dates

3 tablespoons unsalted butter, room temperature

2 eggs, organic preferred

1 teaspoon real vanilla extract

¼ cup raw walnuts, chopped

NOTE: To save yourself the fuss and mess of pureeing the prunes for this recipe, consider buying a packaged version. (We use organic baby food!)

PREHEAT THE OVEN TO 325 DEGREES.
GREASE AN 8 X 8-INCH BAKING PAN.

In a small bowl, combine the cocoa, flour, and salt. Set aside.

In a processor or an electric mixer, blend the prunes, dates, butter, eggs, and vanilla, until smooth.

Add the flour mixture and blend well. Stir in the walnuts.

Using a spatula, spread the batter into pan evenly. Bake until the edges feel dry to the touch but the center appears fudgy, about 20 to 25 minutes. Do not over bake.

Remove from the oven and let cool in pan before cutting. For maximum moistness, store squares in an airtight container.

YIELD: SIXTEEN 2-INCH SQUARES

HEALTHFUL HINT: The walnuts in this recipe contain the precious essential oils that help the immune system cool inflammation.

Hot and Cold Beverages

Frozen Banana-Pineapple Daiquiri

Citrus Sipper

Peach and Ginger Shake

Bloody-Good-For-You Cocktail

Berry Berry Good Smoothie

Minty Yogurt Lassi

Tropical Tea Punch Bowl

Hot Cinnamon Cider

Ginger-Lemon Brew

Steeped Herbal Teas

Frozen Banana-Pineapple Daiquiri

This luscious drink is also known as The Anti-Inflammatory Daiquiri. The banana, pineapple, and lime juice all have vitamin C, and help to reduce swelling and soreness.

1 ripe banana, peeled and quartered

1 cup fresh pineapple, peeled and cut into chunks, plus 2 pieces for garnish

1 cup unsweetened apple juice

6 to 8 ice cubes

¼ cup fresh lime juice

In a blender, combine the banana, pineapple, apple juice, ice cubes, and lime juice. Blend until smooth.

Pour into daiquiri glasses, and serve with a chunk of pineapple on the rim of the glass.

YIELD: 2 DAIQUIRIS

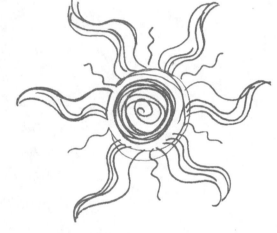

"A daiquiri adds a tropical sparkle to your day"
—Sally Jean

Citrus Sipper

We call this one The Free Radical Quencher! The citrus contains vitamin C and bioflavonoids, which are essential for healthy capillary walls.

Cut the fruit in half and, using an electric citrus juicer, squeeze the oranges and grapefruit into a large container.

Stir well and pour into tall glasses filled with ice and add a straw.

YIELD: 2 SERVINGS

2 Valencia juice oranges

2 tangelo or temple oranges

1 grapefruit

"The health of yourself and your family is a mirror which reflects your intelligence, your efficiency and your cooking methods."

—Adelle Davis

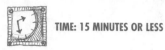
Peach and Ginger Shake

Sweet summer peaches rich in beta carotene, and spicy and fragrant ginger that cools swollen joints—a better combination is hard to find.

2 walnut-sized knobs fresh ginger

2 ripe peaches, pitted and quartered

1 ripe banana, peeled and quartered

1 cup unsweetened apple or peach juice

4 to 6 ice cubes

2 mint sprigs

Using a ginger grater or mini chopper, grate the ginger finely. Gather the pulp with your fingers, and squeeze the juice into a blender. Discard the ginger pulp.

Add the peaches, banana, juice, and ice. Blend until completely smooth.

Pour into beer steins, and place a sprig of mint in each. Serve immediately.

YIELD: 2 SERVINGS

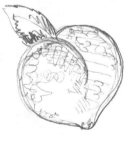

Bloody-Good-For-You Cocktail

Tomatoes are known for their anti-inflammatory properties. They are full of beta carotenoids, which is the plant form of vitamin Λ. So drink up, knowing you're aiding your aches and pains!

In a bottle large enough to fit the ingredients, pour in the tomato and lime juices, soy sauce, pepper, garlic, and a few drops of hot sauce. Place the lid on the bottle and shake well.

Pour into 2 shaped goblets, and slide a stalk of celery into each. Clink the glasses and enjoy!

YIELD: 2 SERVINGS

2 cups fresh or bottled tomato juice (see Note)

1 fresh lime, juiced, about ⅓ cup

1 teaspoon imported soy sauce

Pinch ground black pepper

Pinch garlic powder

Hot sauce

2 young celery stalks with leaves

NOTE: For fresh juice, pass ripe tomatoes through a juicer or puree them in the blender.

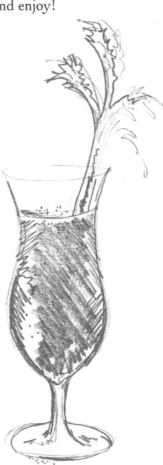

Berry Berry Good Smoothie

Frozen fruit can be stored all year long, making this a refreshing drink even when the summer has long passed.

1 cup fresh or frozen strawberries, green stems removed (see Note)

½ cup fresh or frozen blueberries

¼ to ½ cup fresh or frozen raspberries

1 ripe fresh or frozen banana, peeled and quartered

½ cup unsweetened apple-raspberry or other favorite juice

¼ cup plain yogurt with active cultures

Ice, as needed

NOTE: If you use frozen berries, purchase the fruit-only brands, without sugar or heavy syrups.

In a blender or food processor combine the strawberries, blueberries, raspberries, banana, apple juice, and yogurt. Blend until smooth. (If the fruit is fresh, add several cubes of ice and blend again.)

Serve in tall glasses with a straw.

YIELD: 2 SERVINGS

HEALTHFUL HINT: Bioflavonoids are an essential tool for helping the body regenerate itself in a healthy way They are essential for maintaining healthy capillary walls and metabolizing vitamin C, which is needed for building connective tissue. Berries, onions, citrus fruit (membranes and pith) and kasha all contain bioflavonoids.

Minty Yogurt Lassi

Yogurt with active cultures contributes fresh flora to your intestines and helps with the digestion and assimilation of nutrients.

I n a blender combine the yogurt, mint, honey, and salt. Blend until smooth.

Half fill 2 wine glasses with ice, and pour the lassi over. Serve immediately.

YIELD: 2 SERVINGS

2 cups plain yogurt with active cultures

10 fresh mint leaves

1 to 2 teaspoons honey

Pinch sea salt

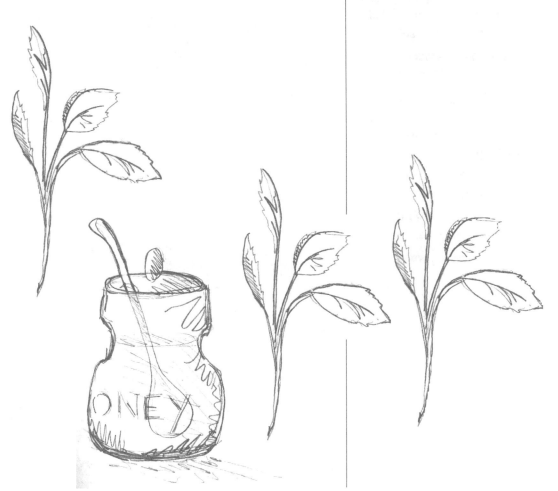

Tropical Tea Punch Bowl

Refreshing and thirst quenching, this Anti-Oxidant Fizz is sensational to serve at your next party. A healthy cocktail which will be a real hit!

This recipe requires frozen pineapple juice (see Note).

2 quarts unsweetened kiwi-strawberry juice or other favorite

2 cups strong brewed herbal fruit tea, caffeine-free

1 pint fresh strawberries, stems removed and sliced

1 orange, organic preferred, quartered and sliced

½ cup fresh or frozen blueberries

½ cup fresh or frozen raspberries

12 frozen unsweetened pineapple juice cubes

1 quart sparkling water

NOTE: Pour unsweetened pineapple juice into an ice cube tray, and allow it to freeze overnight.

In a large punch bowl combine the kiwi-strawberry juice, herbal tea, strawberry and orange slices, blueberries, and raspberries. Add the pineapple ice cubes and sparkling water. Stir and serve.

YIELD: 4½ QUARTS

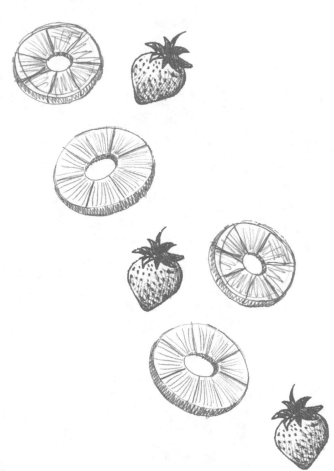

Hot Cinnamon Cider

This crowd pleaser is just what's called for on a winter's afternoon, sitting by the fireside. (The orange pith is full of bioflavonoids.)

In a medium-sized saucepan, combine the cider, cinnamon, cloves, allspice, peppercorn, and orange. Bring to a boil, lower flame and simmer, covered, about 10 minutes.

Place a strainer over another saucepan or teapot. Pour the mulled cider through the strainer.

Arrange 4 beautiful mugs on the counter. Using tongs or a fork, remove the orange quarters and place 2 pieces in each cup. Discard the spices. Pour the hot cider into the cup and serve. Eat the orange pieces, rind and all.

YIELD: 4 SERVINGS

1 quart fresh unsweetened cider

2 cinnamon sticks, broken into pieces

2 whole cloves

2 allspice berries

1 peppercorn

1 orange, organic preferred, cut in eighths

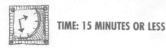
Ginger-Lemon Brew

Yummy and warming, this brew contains many bioflavinoids in the citrus. This Joint Strengthener Drink slows the inflammation response and hastens the healing of athletic injuries.

2 cups unsweetened apple juice or water

4 thin slices fresh ginger

1 lemon, organic preferred

2 teaspoons honey (optional)

I n a medium-sized saucepan heat the apple juice and ginger. Juice the lemon and add, with the rinds, to the juice mixture. Bring to a boil and simmer for 5 minutes.

Strain through a sieve into 2 mugs, and sweeten with honey, if desired.

YIELD: 2 SERVINGS

"Thank God for tea! What would the world do without tea?"

—Sydney Smith

Steeped Herbal Teas

There are such an abundance of caffeine free herbal teas and combinations that we could barely begin to list them here. They are easy to fix, offer a soothing touch, and have quite a friendly nature to your whole body. Start a collection, and enjoy a cup of tea with us!

TO BREW HERBAL TEA: BRING PURIFIED WATER TO A BOIL.

Purified water, 1 cup per person

1 herbal tea bag per person

Honey, lemon, or other flavoring (optional)

Place a tea bag in a favorite cup or several in a ceramic tea pot. (For loose tea, fill a tea ball and place it in a cup or pot.) Pour the boiling water over, and let sit 2 to 5 minutes. (The larger the container, the longer to steep.)

Remove tea bag(s) or ball and discard. Do not reuse tea bags.

Sweeten with honey, a few drops of lemon, or whatever else you prefer.

YIELD: 1 CUP PER PERSON

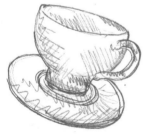
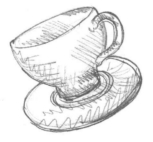
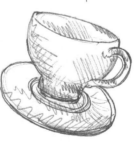
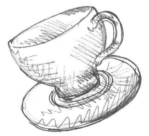

How to Prepare Beans for Cooking

All dried beans need to be sorted and washed. Many beans also need to be soaked before cooking, but there are some that don't. (See the chart on page 196.)

TO SORT: Measure the amount of dry beans that are called for in the recipe. Spill beans onto a flat, surface. Look for stones, cracked beans, and other non-edible items and discard. Place the sorted beans into a large bowl for washing.

TO WASH: Add plenty of purified water to the sorted beans. Swish them around with your hand or a spoon. Drain. Proceed with soaking or cooking, as directed.

TO SOAK: There are two methods for soaking beans:

Long soaking: Add plenty of fresh water to the sorted and washed beans (at least 4 cups of water per 1 cup of dry beans). Set the bowl aside so the beans can soak, uncovered, for 6 to 8 hours, at room temperature. The beans will more than double in size.

Quick soaking: This is also known as the hot soaking method. After sorting and washing the beans, place them in a large saucepan and cover them with 3 or 4 inches of fresh water. Bring the beans to a boil, covered, then lower heat and simmer for 5 minutes. Remove from heat, and allow the beans to sit in the hot water for 2 hours, covered.

TO COOK: Using your hands or a slotted spoon, lift the beans out of the soaking water and place them into a saucepan. (If the beans were quick soaked, remove them to a bowl, and rinse the pot to remove any sand that may have settled on the bottom.) Add the desired amount of liquid (as called for in the recipe). Bring the beans to a boil, covered and proceed with the recipe. Beans are thoroughly cooked when they mash easily when pressed between your fingers or with the tines of a fork.

Which beans need no soaking?: These include green and red lentils, and yellow and green split peas.

Which beans to soak: All other beans need to be soaked in the manner described above. There are numerous varieties of beans, and some common ones are: black, kidney and pinto beans, all the white beans (lima, navy, Great Northern, cannellini), chick-peas, black-eyed peas, etc.

TO ALLEVIATE GASTRIC DISTRESS: Soaking dry beans is especially helpful if you find that eating cooked beans gives you gastric distress. Many people are missing the digestive enzyme alpha-galactosidase which breaks down raffinose sugars that cause gas in the stomach and intestines. There are many things you can do to avoid this problem.

1. Eat beans more frequently. This will help alleviate the gassy problem beans seem to cause, as your digestive tract will store some of the alpha-galactosidase for future use.
2. Change the soaking water one or two times during the 6- to 8- hour soaking period.
3. Rinse the beans after they have been soaked, to remove any remaining raffinose sugars.
4. Do not cook with the bean soaking water.
5. Long soak the beans rather than quick soaking them.
6. Reduce or eliminate (except for yogurt with active cultures) dairy products. Beans seem to be more gaseous when eaten with dairy products.

To add the missing enzyme: Add a few drops of liquid BEANO® to your first bite of beans. This does the trick every time! Call their hotline for a free sample: (800) 257-8650.

STORAGE: Store beans in glass jars for easy identification.

WHY ARE BEANS INCLUDED IN THIS BOOK?

Beans are a good source of plant-based protein, giving you 7 grams in a half cup of cooked beans. Beans are full of vitamins and minerals including zinc, calcium, magnesium, and copper. They are low in calories (about 125 calories per half cup of cooked beans), and are full of soluble fiber, which helps to reduce LDL cholesterol, lower blood pressure, and regulate bowel function. Beans are also rich in potassium, and iron, and these help counter the use of NSAIDs, steroids, and other medications.

When beans are combined with whole

BASIC BEAN COOKING CHART

Bean	Cooking Time
Chick peas	1½ - 2½ hours
Black beans	1½ hours
Black-eyed peas	35 minutes
Cannellini beans	1 hour
Great Northern beans	45 minutes
Green lentils*	45 minutes
Kidney beans	50 minutes
Lima beans, small	45 minutes
Lima beans, large	1 hour
Navy beans	40 minutes
Pinto beans	45 minutes
Red lentils*	20 minutes
Split peas*	1½ hours
*requires no soaking	

grains or seeds, they become a complete protein with a full complement of amino acids, providing a higher amount of useable protein than when using just the beans alone.

More about beans: Beans can be cooked in various methods, which include boiling, baking, pressure cooking, or a slow cooker. Never cook the following beans in a pressure cooker: green and yellow split peas, and red or green lentils, since these tend to foam and clog the pressure cooker vent.

Do not add salt, sweeteners, fats, tomatoes, or vinegar while beans are cooking, since this will harden the bean's skin and lengthen the cooking process. If none of these ingredients have been added and the beans are still not softening within recommended cooking time, they could be old. If this is the case, puree the semi-cooked beans and then continue cooking them for another 10 to 15 minutes (or discard the beans and start over). When making bean salad, the beans can be salted after half of the cooking process has passed, to keep them from falling apart and becoming mushy.

Beans are now available in jars and they taste much better than the ones in cans—and have no preservatives and less added salt.

Whole Grain Facts

TO WASH: Measure the amount of grain needed for the recipe and pour it into a saucepan. Cover them with plenty of purified water (3 to 4 inches) and swish the grains around with your hand or a spoon to loosen any dust and inedible fibers.

TO DRAIN: Have a sieve handy (a colander's holes are too large). Drain the grain, return to the saucepan, and cook as directed.

TO COOK: Cook grains according to the recipe instructions, adding the suggested amount of liquid, cover and proceed with the recipe. (See chart on page 200.)

Which grains need no washing? Pasta, kasha, bulghur, couscous, and any grain that has been cut, flaked, broken or rolled, such as steel cut oats and bulgur wheat.

Grains that need washing: Rice (brown, wehani, basmati, wild, etc.), barley, millet, quinoa, and any other whole grain.

How to store whole grains: Store whole grains in covered glass jars, for easy identification. Add a bay leaf, to keep moths from hatching and infesting.

*Why are whole grains suggested
in this book?*

Whole grains, with their bran and germ intact, contain all the major nutrient groups; carbohydrates, protein, fats, vitamins, minerals, and fiber. They are a rich source of insoluble fiber, important fats, and B vitamins. When combined with a complementary protein such as beans or seeds, they also become a complete protein, with all the needed amino acids. Whole grains are complex carbohydrates.

When whole grains are refined, twenty two essential nutrients including the fiber are removed. Four to six nutrients are replaced, and this depleted food is labeled as "enriched". It is no longer a complex carbohydrate. The bran contains the fiber and the B vitamins, and removing the germ depletes the essential oils and fat-soluble vitamins E and K. The process of refining a grain leaves the starchy, carbohydrate part only, which is called the endosperm. For example, white rice is the endosperm only. It is derived from brown rice that has the bran and germ polished off. Whole wheat and white flour follow this same pattern. The refined counterparts are nutritionally inferior to their whole grain beginnings.

According to the Composition of Foods published by the USDA, when brown rice is compared with white, brown has 12 percent more protein, 33 percent more calcium, 5 times more vitamin B1, 67 percent more vitamin B2, 3 times more niacin, and 2½ times as much potassium and iron. It has 100 percent more vitamin E, as there is none left in white rice.

Whole grains are osteoarthritis fighters. They contain antioxidants, bioflavonoids, and counter the use of NSAIDs, steroids, and other medications.

What about pasta? There are many whole grain pastas on the market that taste great and can be used interchangeably with recipes that call for white flour or semolina pasta. These pastas now come in a variety of shapes and forms. Look for whole wheat, buckwheat, brown rice, spelt, and corn. The Japanese also have udon noodles, which are made from whole wheat, and soba made from buckwheat flour. Stay away, from artichoke and spinach pastas, since these are made with a base of white flour and are missing the important nutrients needed for arthritic joints. Semolina flour is refined durum wheat and is also to be avoided in its refined state. Read labels to be assured that the flour is a whole grain.

A word about barley: The bran and germ of barley is fused to the endosperm. They are usually ground off, leaving a small, round, white pearl. This barley is known as pearled barley. This is the variety that one finds in the grocery store. A better quality barley is one that does not have all of the bran and germ removed, is somewhat oval, is tan or brown, and is found in the natural food store. It is often called pearled barley, as well. There is also whole barley which is dark brown, fully oval and requires 4 to 6 hours of soaking before cooking. The recipes in this book call for the slightly pearled variety of barley, found in the natural food store.

BASIC WHOLE GRAIN COOKING CHART

Whole Grain (1 cup)	Liquid	Cooking Time
Barley, slightly pearled	2 cups	1 hour
Brown rice, long grain	1½ cups	55 minutes
Brown rice, short grain	2 cups	55 minutes
Bulgur*	1½ cups, boiling	10 minutes
Cornmeal*	4 to 5 cups (cold)	45 minutes
Couscous*	1½ cups, boiling	10 minutes
Kasha (buckwheat)*	2 cups, boiling	10 minutes
Millet	2 cups	35 minutes
Oatmeal*	2 cups	20 minutes
Oats, steel cut*	2 cups	30 minutes
Pasta, whole grain*	1 - 2 quarts	as per package
Quinoa	2 cups	15 minutes
Wild rice	3 cups	1 hour

*requires no washing

Updating your ingredients

AGAR: A vegetarian source of gelatin that is used commercially as a stabilizer, thickener, binding agent, and emulsifier. Most coastal areas have used agar and other sea vegetables for centuries. It is available in bars, flakes, or powder. Agar can be substituted for gelatin but has stronger setting properties, so less of it is required.

BACON: On occasion, this meat treat is wonderful to add flavor to a dish. Commercial bacon and cured meats are processed with sodium nitrite or nitrate, a food additive used to stabilize the pink or red color in meats, enhance flavor, and protect against bacterial growth.

When heated, nitrites chemically react with amine compounds to form nitrosamines, which can be carcinogenic. This kind of bacon also contains BHT, a preservative, various sugars (white, brown, and/or corn syrup), and an excess amount of salt. If bacon or cured meats are used, we recommend the kind found in natural markets.

BEANS: See "How to Prepare Beans" page 195.

BREAD CRUMBS, WHOLE GRAIN: These are missing the hydrogenated fats, chemical flavoring, and preservatives. Available in the natural food store or make your own using stale or toasted whole grain bread, crackers, or bread sticks that are pulverized in the blender or food processor.

Store extras in the freezer or refrigerator.

BROWN RICE: According to the Composition of Foods published by the USDA, when brown rice is compared with white, brown has 12 percent more protein, 33 percent more calcium, 5 times more vitamin B1, 67 percent more vitamin B2, 3 times more niacin, and 2 1/2 times as much potassium and iron. It has 100 percent more vitamin E, as there is none left in white rice.

Therefore, to get the full range of nutrition and healing properties from your food, choose brown over white rice whenever possible.

BUTTER: Unsalted or sweet butter has a delicate flavor. Store several unsalted sticks of butter in the freezer (for up to 6 months), and one in the refrigerator for daily use (about 2 weeks). Butter is excellent for baking because it is stable at high temperatures and has the best taste.

BUTTERMILK: A tangy by-product of buttermaking, it is thicker than milk. Also see yogurt.

CONSERVES: Naturally sweetened, all-fruit jams made from good quality fruit of optimum ripeness, without the use of added sweetener.

CORNMEAL, HIGH-LYSINE: High-lysine cornmeal contains the amino acid lysine that is missing in commercial cornmeal. This maintains its sweet and nutty taste for a longer time than its commercial counterpart.

DEHYDRATED VEGETABLES: Garlic and onion are the most common in this category, and are found in flake and powder form. If using the fresh garlic or onions causes too much digestive discomfort, dried can add plenty of flavor to your recipes. Look for those without additives or preservatives. Also see herbs.

EGGS, ORGANIC: The chickens that lay these eggs are free of antibiotics and added hormones that can burden your system. When the chickens are free-range, they eat a more natural diet, and tend to have thicker shells and a richer flavor.

All eggs provide a good source of high-quality protein, plus iron, zinc, and vitamins A, B2, D, E, and K. All of these nutrients are recommended to halt, reverse, and cure osteoarthritis.

FLOUR: There are two whole wheat flours available. One is whole wheat pastry flour, ground from soft wheat and best when used for cookies, cakes, quick breads, pancakes, and other pastries. The other is whole wheat flour, which is derived from hard wheat and better when used for yeast bread. They can be used interchangeably when called for in a roux or sauce. Most other grains are available in flour form, and they can be experimented with for taste and texture preferences.

GELATIN: An odorless, tasteless, and colorless jelling agent. It is a pure protein derived from beef and veal bones, cartilage, and other tissues. Granulated gelatin is the most common form of unsweetened commercial gelatin on the market. 1 envelope will gel 2 cups of liquid. Soak it first in cold liquid for 3 to 5 minutes to soften the granules so they will dissolve evenly when heated. Gelatin helps to soothe inflamed joints.

GHEE: This is clarified butter which has had the milk solids removed. It can be used on a higher flame than butter or oil, without smoking. Organic ghee is available already prepared, or melt your own butter on a low heat and then refrigerate until cool. Separate the fat from the milk solids and store.

GRAINS: See *Whole Grain Facts* page 199.

GRAINS, CREAM OF: Finely ground cereals made from wheat, rye, rice, corn (grits), or buckwheat, that cook in 5 minutes.

HERBS AND SPICES: Not all herbs and spices are bottled the same. Commercial herbs and spices are frequently mixed with preservatives to maintain freshness. We prefer the varieties without these additives. Many herbs and spices are now available organically grown.

HERBAL SALT: Flavorful herbs added to sea salt. Look for brands without hydrolyzed vegetable protein, hydrogenated oils, sugar, monosodium glutamate (MSG), preservatives, and free-flowing chemicals. Herbal salt is a little less salty than sea salt alone, and can be used interchangeably.

JUICE BOTTLED: We recommend juice that is 100% fruit juice, unfiltered, and without preservatives or refined sugars. These are usually cloudy, contain some fiber, and pectin, and have more nutrients than the clear varieties. Many commercial juices are made from fruit purees, concentrates, or nectars, which have added water and/or sugars. If the juice is labeled drink, cocktail, or punch, they contain very little fruit juice and a great deal of sugar, as well as artificial flavors and colorings.

KASHA: Kasha is dry-roasted buckwheat. It is available milled in fine, medium, and coarse forms, but the unmilled kind is the best tasting. Its natural shape, when whole, is triangular. Unroasted buckwheat is a creamy white color, and once roasted it has a brown color and is called kasha. Since it is pre-toasted, this grain does not get washed before cooking.

LEMON AND LIME JUICE: Bottled juices are a great convenience and can save labor and hand strength. These juices have lots of vitamin C and taste best when freshly squeezed. For most of us, this isn't practical and requires a lot of citrus fruits. There are several bottled brands without preservatives and other chemicals; organic is available, too.

LEMON, LIME, AND ORANGE ZEST: When a recipe calls for the rind of the lemon, it is preferable to use organic citrus to avoid the anti-mold agents and other chemicals that are sprayed on the fruit before and after harvest.

LIVER, ORGANIC: A wide range of vitamins and minerals are contained in this organ meat, including vitamins A, K, and B12, folic acid, niacin, selenium, zinc, and iron. Liver from an animal raised on clean feed with minimal environmental contamination is what we recommend.

MAPLE SYRUP: Real maple syrup is made from the sap of the maple tree that is boiled until the water has evaporated and maple sugars have concentrated. It is *not* the same as maple-flavored syrup, which is produced from less expensive syrups such as corn syrup and artificial maple flavor and color. Real maple syrup has many minerals including calcium, potassium, manganese, magnesium, phosphorus, and iron.

MISO PASTE: A fermented bean paste made by cooked soybeans and/or other beans with a culture, salt, and water, and fermenting the mixture for several months to 2 years. Use miso in soups or sauces instead of bouillon or as stock when diluted with water. It can also be used instead of salt in salad dressing, sauce, or to flavor beans, grains or stew. The taste is similar to soy sauce.

MUSHROOMS: Available in dried and fresh forms, they are a delight for both taste and nutrient value. Mushrooms can be added to almost any dish. Soak **dry mushrooms** in purified water for 15 to 20 minutes. Squeeze excess water, from them and cook. *Fresh mushrooms* need a quick rinse in water to remove any peat moss from the growing and packaging process. Do not soak fresh mushrooms in water, or their flavor will dilute.

Cepes have a nutty flavor and strong mushroom taste. They are also known as porcini. *Chanterelles* are known for their apricot-like aroma and taste.

Buttons are cultivated white mushrooms with a mild and earthy flavor.

Enoki have a long thin stem with a tiny, snow white cap. They are very mild tasting and have an appealing crunchy texture.

Morels have a rich, smoky, nutty, and woodsy flavor. Dried morels are more intense tasting than fresh ones.

Oyster mushrooms have a robust flavor with a slightly peppery taste that dissipates when cooked.

Portobello is a large, dark brown mushroom, and when sautéed, has a robust and meaty taste and texture.

Shiitake have a distinct aroma and taste. The dry ones have a chewy texture, while fresh shiitake are more mild in taste and texture. The stems are best when used in a stock and then discarded.

Tree ear or *cloud ear* mushrooms are available in the dried form and expand 5 to 6 times after soaking. They impart little flavor, but add a crunchy texture.

OIL: A good vegetable oil is one labeled "extra virgin," "unrefined," or "expeller pressed." It should appear somewhat dark and be close to the color, taste, and smell of the raw ingredient. Refined oils are "solvent-extracted" from the source seed or nut by grinding the ingredient and soaking it in a chemical solvent and later boiling most of it off. They are then treated until they're transparent, giving them no taste or color. These oils are highly refined and are not recommended. Also see hydrogenated oils.

OIL, FLAXSEED: This oil is high in omega-3 fatty acids, which are special polyunsaturated oils that are very beneficial for osteoarthritis, coronary health, and brain growth and development. They help to reduce inflammation. Fatty meat fish are also a source of omega-3s.

OIL, HYDROGENATED OR PARTIALLY HYDROGENATED: Liquid oil is chemically altered into a solid state by pumping hydrogen atoms into the unsaturated fat—obliterating any benefits it had as a vegetable oil. Many scientists believe that hydrogenated oils may be more damaging than regular saturated fats. Margarine and vegetable shortening are in this category.

OLIVE OIL, EXTRA VIRGIN: Produced from the first pressing of ripe olives, this oil contains oil-soluble vitamins, lecithin, essential fatty acids, phytohormones, some minerals, and antioxidants that act like preservatives, such as vitamin E, that keep the oil from going rancid. Store in a dark bottle, away from light and heat, and keep only small quantities unrefrigerated for daily use.

PASTA: Use whole grain pastas made with whole wheat, brown rice, corn, or buckwheat flours. See *Whole Grain Facts*, page 199.

PASTA, FLAVORED: Artichoke, spinach, tomato, and squid ink pastas are all made with a base of refined white or semolina flour, which have had the nutrients and fiber removed. They are inferior to whole grain pastas.

PURIFIED WATER: See *water*.

SALAD DRESSING: Bottled dressings and dips are full of sugar, salt, refined oils, chemicals, and preservatives. Look for brands that use better quality oils such as extra virgin olive oil, and are made without refined sugars, chemicals, or preservatives. (Hint: Add a few tablespoons of water to dips to create a creamy and delicious salad dressing.)

SALT: Sea salt is solar dried sea water that has no chemical additives, sugar, or aluminum. Commercial salt is processed using steam heat, under pressure up to 1200 degrees and then it is flash cooled to produce crystals. Aluminum is added to prevent caking, potassium iodide is added to provide iodine, and then dextrose is used to hold the iodine molecule, keeping it from being unstable.

SEA VEGETABLES: In general these are a rich source of easy-to-digest proteins, vitamins,

and minerals such as vitamins A, B, B12, C, and E, and calcium, phosphorous, magnesium, iron, and iodine. Also see *agar*.

SOBA NOODLES: Made from 100 percent buckwheat flour or a mixture of buckwheat and wheat flours. Soba can be served chilled or hot. Their shape is like that of spaghetti, although they taste nothing like it. Soba tastes better with nontomato sauces, such as our Satay Sauce.

SOY SAUCE: Good quality soy sauce is naturally brewed in wooden kegs and made with water, soy beans, sea salt, and sometimes wheat. The imported and natural soy sauces may be labeled as real soy sauce, tamari, or shoyu—and they taste much better too. The commercially produced product is made from refined soy meal which is treated with hydrochloric acid, heated, and then sodium carbonate is added to neutralize the acid. This type has additives including caramel color, corn syrup, BHT and other preservatives, and has never been fermented.

SPICES: See *herbs and spices*.

SUGAR, WHITE: A highly refined product made from sugar cane or sugar beets. During processing, fiber, vitamins, minerals, amino acids, and trace elements are stripped. Since refined sugar is lacking fiber, it is absorbed into the blood stream too quickly, causing the pancreas and adrenal glands to overreact. This can lead to irritability and fatigue. Refined sugar contains no nutrients other than simple carbohydrates, but requires some vitamins and minerals to be metabolized. Thus, it takes nutrients away from the body's other needs, such as cell growth, protein synthesis, etc. Those with arthritis cannot afford to lose any vitamins or minerals, which are needed to mend joints and cartilage. It is recommended to avoid sugar and products containing it.

TAHINI: A very versatile ground sesame paste that has the amino acids to complement beans, being rich in methionine and low in lysine, of which beans have the opposite. It is suitable to use tahini on toast and in puddings, spreads, dips, salad dressings, soups, desserts, and any other place you can think of.

UDON NOODLES: These are Japanese noodles made from whole wheat flour and/or brown rice flour. Udon can be served hot or cold, and tastes great with tomato sauce. It is shaped like narrow fettuccini.

VANILLA EXTRACT: A favorite flavoring for all sorts of sweets. Real vanilla extract is made from vanilla beans aged in alcohol and is free of sugars, caramel coloring, and other additives. Vanillin is derived from the waste products of the wood processing industry and it is recommended that this product never be used. Some manufacturers produce a non-alcoholic, vegetable oil-based extract. This, and the real extract, are available in the natural food store.

WATER: Our bodies are made up of approx-imately 70 percent water, which is involved in transporting nutrients throughout the body and nearly every other body process, including absorption, circulation, and carrying out waste material. It is important to drink and cook with quality water.

WATER, PURIFIED: In the 1970s, studies conducted by the Environmental Protection Agency revealed a high level of heavy metals and many chemical contaminants in household water. These findings led to standards to limit the number of chemicals, pesticides, bacteria, radioactivity, and turbidity. Although these standards have been set, they are not enforced nationally, and as new compounds and chemicals make their way into the water supply, regulation and testing becomes very difficult. Chlorine, phosphates, sodium aluminates, lime, and other chemicals are added to the water in order to reach the minimum standard. Many of these chemicals have been found to lower the amount of nutrients your body absorbs and may have other toxic side effects. Pollutants, such as fertilizers, insecticides, and lead from automobile and factory exhausts are washed into the surface water. It is for these reasons we recommend purified water so the nutrients you take and get in your food will be used for healing your arthritis.

WHOLE WHEAT PASTA: Made from durum wheat that has the bran and germ intact. It has a rich, nutty flavor and is more filling than white or semolina pasta. It is much more nutritionally advantageous than the refined pastas commonly served. Also see *Whole Grain Facts*, (page 199).

YOGURT: Plain yogurt with living cultures has had the active bacteria added after the milk is pasteurized and the yogurt is made, so they are still living when you eat the yogurt. This type of yogurt provides protein, calcium, and beneficial cultures which inhibit harmful bacteria and promotes bet- ter digestion and elimination. The beneficial cultures are lactobacillus bulgaricus, bifidus, lactobacillus acidophilus, and others. Those who normally have difficulty digesting milk and milk products may have better results using yogurt. In recipes, you can substitute yogurt for milk, cream, buttermilk, mayonnaise, or sour cream.

Mail Order Sources

Bandon Sea-Pack: Salmon and tuna. 800-255-4370

Beano® Hotline and free sample: 800-257-8650

Bioforce of America: Herbal sea salt and teas. 800-445-8802

Broken Arrow Ranch: Wild Game. 800-962-4263

Diamond Organics: Organic Fruits and Vegetables. 800-922-2396

D'Artagnan: Chicken, turkey, and game. 800-327-8246

Natural Beef Farms: Beef, chicken, lamb, pork, bacon, keilbasa, sausage. 703-631-8705

Organic Valley: Organic cheeses, butter, chicken, pork, beef, and lamb. Call for distributor sources. 608-625-2602

Silver Creek Farm: Fresh produce, lamb, chicken, turkey, and blueberries, and certified organic beef. 330-569-3487

Timber Crest Farms: Unsulphured dry fruits, sundried tomatoes, fruit butters. 707-433-8251

Walnut Acres: A grocery store by mail featuring whole grains and cereals, beans, soup mixes, condiments, and more. 800-433-3998

Vermont Country Maple Naturals: Maple syrup. 800-528-7021

A good source for other mail order foods is:

Green Groceries—A mail order Guide to Organic Foods, by Jeanne Heifetz (HarperCollins, 1992)

GOOD GRIPS household and outdoor products. 800-545-4411

Sammons Preston. The Preferred Source of Rehabilitation Professionals. 800-323-1745

Index